THE ART OF THERAPY

A PRACTICAL HOW TO GUIDE FOR THERAPISTS

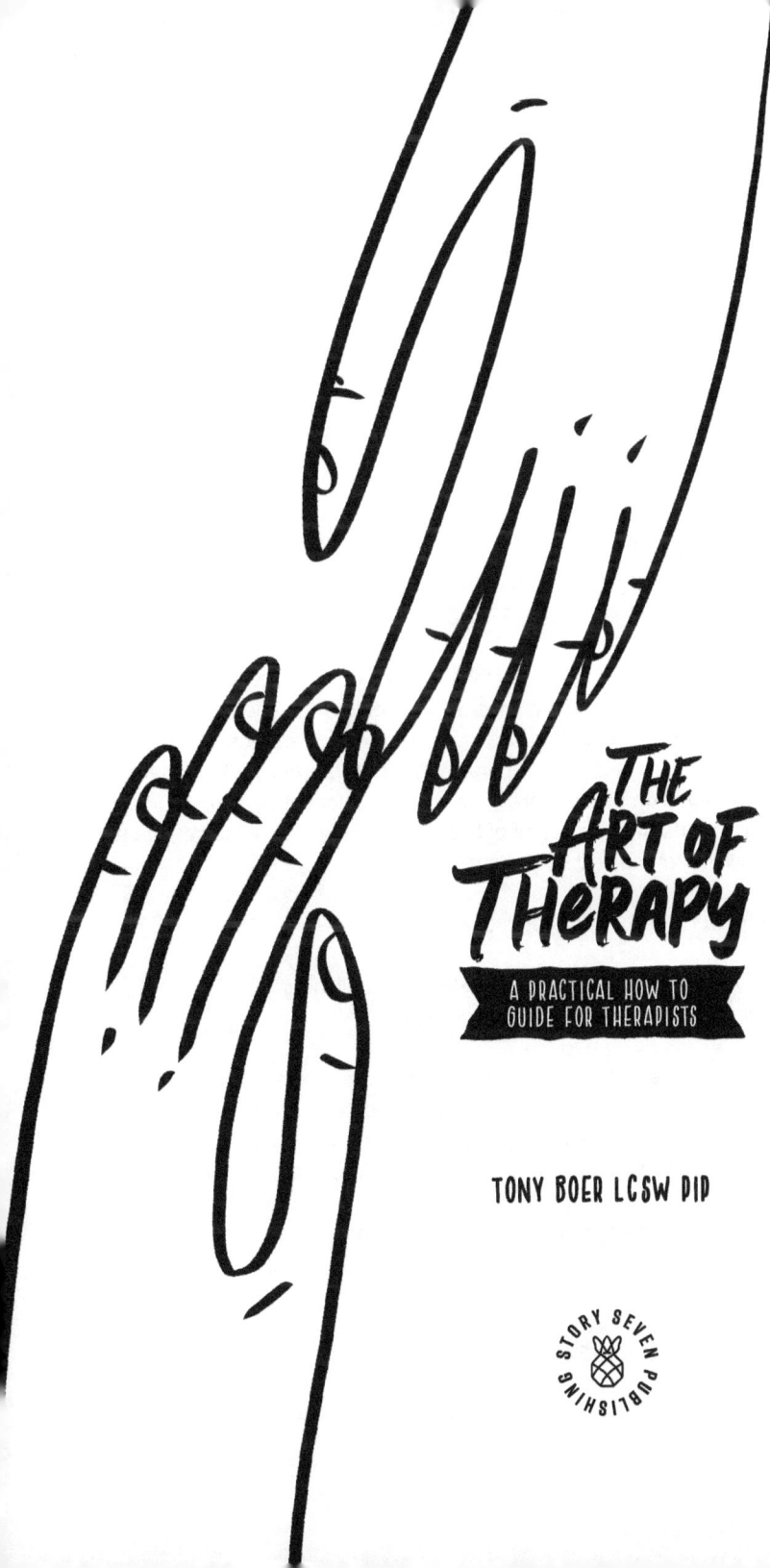

THE ART OF THERAPY

A PRACTICAL HOW TO GUIDE FOR THERAPISTS

TONY BOER LCSW DIP

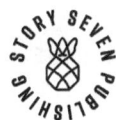

STORY SEVEN PUBLISHING

DEDICATION

This book is dedicated to all the people who have sat across from me on the couch teaching me so many valuable insights.

Thank you.

TABLE OF CONTENTS

Section I:

ESTABLISHING A CONNECTION

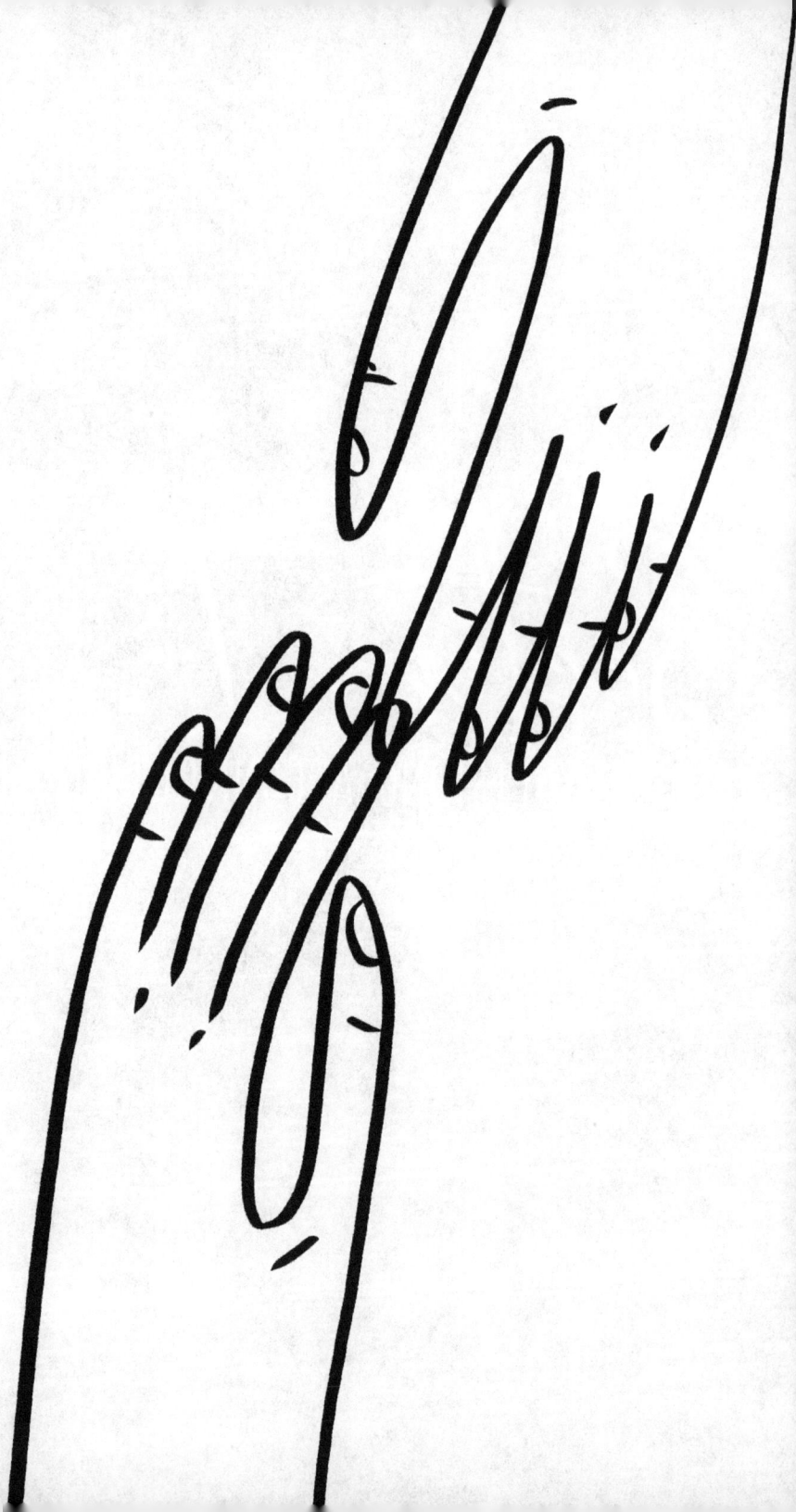

Goal of the Book

GOAL OF THE BOOK

My goal in writing this book is to help new therapists identify how to "do" therapy—not from a theoretical standpoint but a practical one. Seasoned therapists may read this and go, "Duh," but new therapists often feel lost and overwhelmed when they begin their careers. I have supervised a number of new therapists over the years and have found myself repeating some of the same stories and concepts. As you will see, I tend to look at themes, and one common theme I notice with new therapists is that they know the theoretical approach to a problem but lack training on how to get to a spot that allows them to begin to use their knowledge effectively.

New therapists facing case studies can do an excellent job reading symptoms on paper to correctly diagnosing a patient. They can state that the person has depression and would benefit from cognitive behavioral therapy, in which the therapist should challenge the patient's negative thoughts and addresses the faulty core beliefs. Perfect! Sounds great.

Then I ask the new therapist, "How are you going to do that," or "Okay. So what are you going to say in your session to your client?" That is when the lost look arrives. I follow with:

- "What type of mood or environment do you want to set in the sessions?"
- "What is your goal for Session 1?"
- "How are you going to get all the case study info? Are you going to ask a bunch of questions?"
- "Are you going to let them lead, or are you going to lead?"

It very quickly becomes evident that the practical stuff has not been practiced enough, or even thought about at all. This is unfortunate, as setting the tone and mood of a therapy session can lead to success or failure. A successful therapy encounter often is more dependent on how the session "feels" than what is actually said. If you do not get started on the right foot, you will never get the chance to do your 'theoretical" stuff, as the client will not be coming back! So much happens outside of the actual treatment part of therapy, and it is essential for therapists to know how to manage and handle that aspect.

Therapy is part science and theory and part art. My aim with this book is to aid with the art area of therapy. This provides a challenge, as I am trying to describe feelings, moods, and attitudes that are difficult to qualify or quantify. You can describe a painting to another person, but allowing that person to actually experience it is way more powerful and moving. Or for sports fans, would you rather watch a game on TV or see it in person? You can see fans cheering loudly on TV, but when you are there to witness the ups and downs of your team losing before pulling it out at the end, it is a completely different experience. This book is trying to help you "be there" with me in therapy sessions, so when you are actually in your own sessions you can be beneficial to your clients. This is the best way I can explain the art of therapy with all of its subtleties and intricacies. Some of the most powerful moments in a therapy session involve noticing your client's facial reactions or their shifts in body language when you or someone else enters the room. If you can pick up on that feeling and express it out loud, that moment can lead to a breakthrough that has nothing to do with theories or knowledge about depression or anxiety.

Human connection is powerful. You must connect with your clients before you can do any of the "work" of therapy. I argue that the connection is THE MOST IMPORTANT THING you will do in therapy. You will not see a lot about it in textbooks, as art is hard to qualify, measure, and prove effective. You will see lots of numbers in therapy regarding effectiveness and success rates. Insurance companies will not reimburse because you have a great connection. They will not pay you if you report, "We get along nicely." They will only reimburse you if you employ a proven theory with clear, measureable, and reproducible goals. You will need a theory to practice and make a living, and there are necessary hoops you need to jump through to keep you on task and hold you accountable. These practices provide great protections for clients to make sure they are getting help. However, none of your services will provide benefit if you do not connect with your client.

This book is certainly not intended as a replacement for any particular theory, supervision, or consultation. My material is additive to what is in your textbooks. I have a certain theoretical orientation that guides my therapy. New therapists often ask me how to approach a situation or to recommend a right way to handle something. Before I answer, I ask them to tell them me about their plans, theories and approaches, and I find those can often lead to similar results. Whether you have a cognitive behavioral approach, an object relations approach, or a strengths approach, I will ask you the same questions: "Why you are doing what you are doing?" and "Do you have a plan and goal?" If you do have a plan and goal, great! If you don't, it's time to go back to the client and make a better connection so you can learn what the client wants to achieve and help the client achieve success. How you get there can take a bunch of different paths.

I hope that this book will provide you with some insight, provoke some new thinking, and help you appreciate the art and connection of therapy.

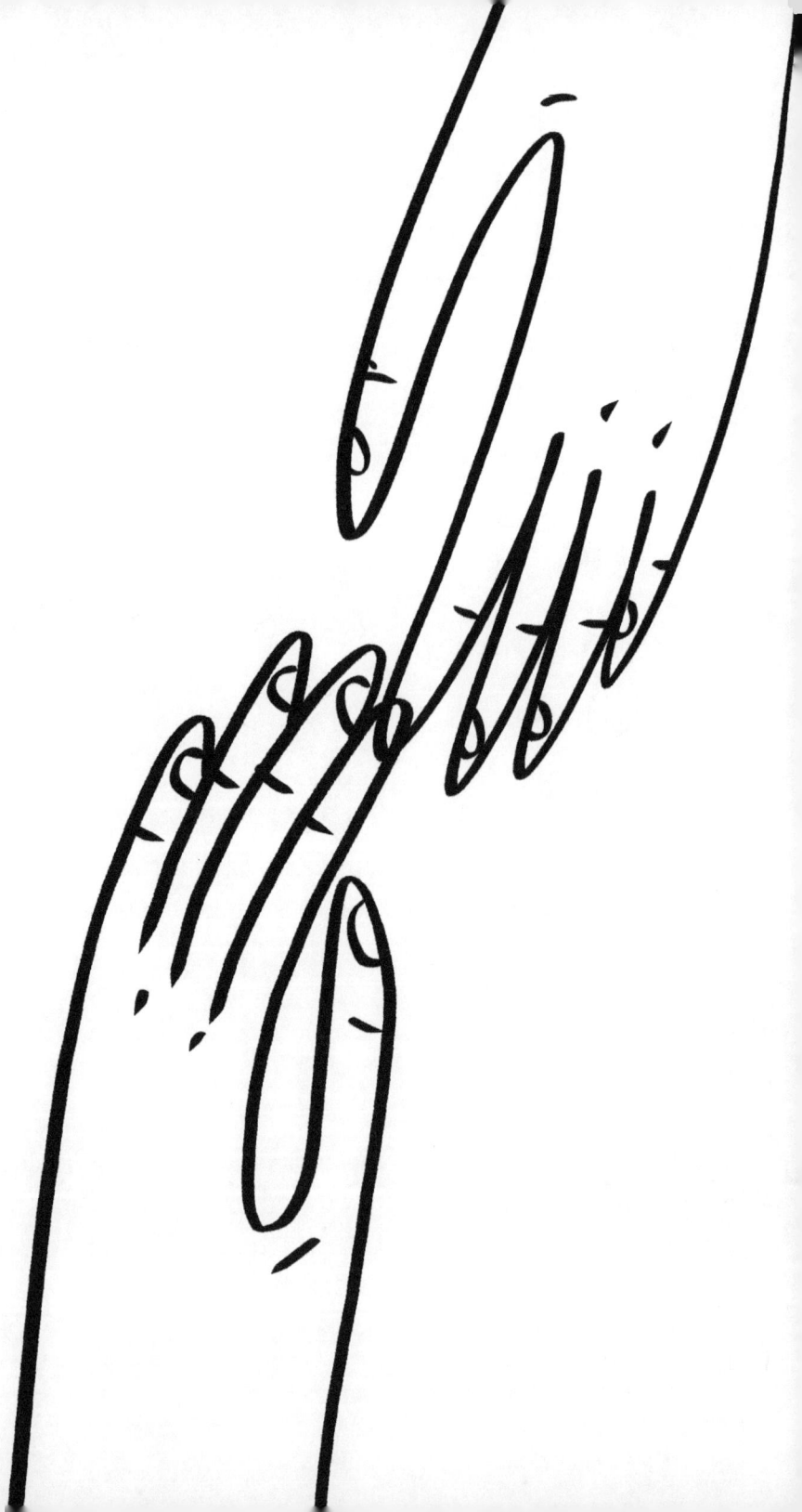

SECTION I: PART II

My Approach

MY APPROACH

My suggestions in this book aren't based on scientific research or tried-and-true principles. They are based on my experiences in therapy with the techniques that tend to lead to success and those that have fell short. My approach remains a work on progress.

Working with people has taught me a lot of things. I am privileged to hear story after story of people's trials and tribulations. People are amazing, resilient, and strong. When I first heard that we are made in God's image, I have often wondered what that means. You can look around the world and see people of all shapes and sizes, but you'll also notice so many different personality types—Type A people who are organized and structured, right-brained people who are articulate and creative, easy-going people, easily frustrated people, conservative people, liberal people, nice people, mean people, etc. You'll meet awesome people you want to be around, and, unfortunately, people that you do not want to be around!

So where is God's image in all of this? I am beginning to think that part of it comes from our desire to be loved and accepted. Everyone I have ever met either in counseling or in my personal life wants to feel loved and valued. Love is part of the image of God we carry around. From a theological standpoint, I think that is why we are made to praise God—to make him smile! God likes to be loved as well, and that may be part of the reason he gave us freewill.

I know this may sound a little cheesy, but it is so powerful. My personal belief is that our desire to be loved and accepted comes from God's ultimate unconditional love for us. To live in God's image, we have this need to love and be loved. I am sure there is more to the "made in God's image" piece, and I would never want to say I know what God is thinking or doing. But I recognize something consistently in people that despite being clouded by sin and corruption, humanity appears to be based on something bigger.

Why this little sermon about God's image? I want to lay the ground-work for the importance and power of connection. This desire to feel loved and valued exists in all of us, and the need to have it addressed is central to how people act in the world. You will hear it expressed in a variety of terms and phrases in the coming pages: acceptance, love, value, feeling important, know-ing you matter, your purpose, your meaning of why you do what you do, safety, security—all encompassing the same concept. Addressing this need for love is central to helping people, and creating a connection with someone is another way of saying, "I love you" and "I find value in you."

People often ask me questions such as, "How do you sit and listen to people complain for hours on end," or "How do you deal with all the hurt that people are sharing?" Or they say, "I could never do your job! You probably have heard some crazy stories," or, "How do you deal with people who just are mean and difficult?"

A lot of those statements hold some truth. It is exhausting to hear people fight, and it is not a good day when a marriage dies on the couch in front of you. It is not a good day when a child tells you about years of abuse. It is not a good day when a child tells you they are in their ninth foster home, and then asks if you can just take him home so he does not have to keep going from family to family. It is not a good day when a person tells you with conviction in their heart that there is no reason to be alive.

This is just a small sample of the many hurts expressed during sessions, and I know that there are many more that have never dared to be spoken. So if this is the bad side of being a therapist, there has to be a good side, right? Most definitely! Surely, ER doctors don't do what they do to witness death; their reward is witness saving and healing. We, as therapists, must cultivate that same perspective by staying in the moment and building connection with people. I don't see a couple fighting on the couch. I see two people passionately telling each other the extent of their hurt. If they are hurt, it means they care. When I get them on my couch and they are fighting and hurting each other, I try to slow things down and ask them why they are here in my office? Sometimes it takes a while to get there, but eventually we hear the truth. Here is an example:

> **Husband:** (After they have been telling me how mad they are and it is gradually getting louder in my office.) "See, this is how she talks. She never listens to what I say."

Wife: "I don't listen?! I am telling you things all the time that you never do. You don't listen and I can't take it anymore."

Husband: "Well, I am done."

Wife: "Done? What do you mean, 'done'? You are going to bail now? Of course you are. You care only about yourself?"

Husband: "That is what you keep saying. So what is the point? You won't change.

(This happens a lot, and yes, this is not fun.)

Therapist: "Who set up this appointment?"

Wife: "I did. I have been asking him for years to come to counseling and he refuses."

Therapist: Why?"

Wife: "I don't like how things are and I am so mad at him."

Therapist: Why are you so mad at him?"

Wife: "I don't really know. I just don't like it when we are yelling at each other. I thought things would be better. They used to be better. I miss how things used to be."

Therapist: "What do you miss?"

Wife: "I miss him."

Therapist: (to husband): "Why did you come?"

Husband: "She made me."

Therapist: "She did? How did she do that?"

Husband: "She said if I did not come she was going to leave?"

Therapist: "You don't want her to leave?"

Husband: "Well no!"

Therapist: "Why don't you want her to leave? She never listens to you and makes your life difficult."

Husband: "I don't want to lose her."

Therapist: "Lose her?"

Husband: "I still love her."

It can, of course, take a much longer conversation to get past the anger and hurt, but when you get down to the real stuff and each hurting spouse learns that the other actually cares, that glimmer of hope is powerful. Couples will cry, soften, and even reach out to each other. Now it does not always result in a perfect ending, but giving them a little hope and helping them see that they are loved can be powerful, and this is the "fun" part of therapy. I enjoy helping people turn from the negative to reach for hope and connection, and it makes my job awesome. The ability to help people feel connected, loved, and valuable, even when they are in the darkest spot imaginable, provides more joy than any of the negative that goes with the job. That is the power of connection.

I am going to show you how I build connection with others, but it's important that your approach fit your individuality. Take the concepts I share and mold them to fit your personality. Approaches, especially theoretical ones, often have a number of steps and processes from which you are strongly encouraged not to deviate. My approach calls for the opposite—your personality must shine through. It is essential. Your clients needs somebody (you) not something (theory) with which to connect. Let your personality shine through your therapy. Let your personality shine through your theory.

And that brings us to the next important point—be authentic. Be genuine, as people can identify phoniness and insecurity from a mile away. Be real. If you are trying to teach your clients how to be authentic, you first must show authenticity. This means acknowledging what you can and can't do, and acknowledging what you know and don't know. I often say, "I have no idea," in therapy sessions. And when a client replies with something like, "Well, I thought you were the expert!" I respond, "I never said that, and I am most certainly not an expert on you! I trust that you know you better than I do!"

We will go over these concepts in more detail, but it is first helpful to look at the bigger picture. We don't take off on long trips before looking at the map on our phones, and we shouldn't jump into therapeutic details before first establishing a connection and looking at some of the common themes of a client's problems or struggles. By identifying a theme to those issues, we are able to ascertain a general direction toward help. Clients often can't see the forest for the trees, but they can list their struggles. If you can connect with a client and then classify their struggles into a common theme, then (and only then) can you start to identify a treatment plan that brings in your theories and problem-solving approaches.

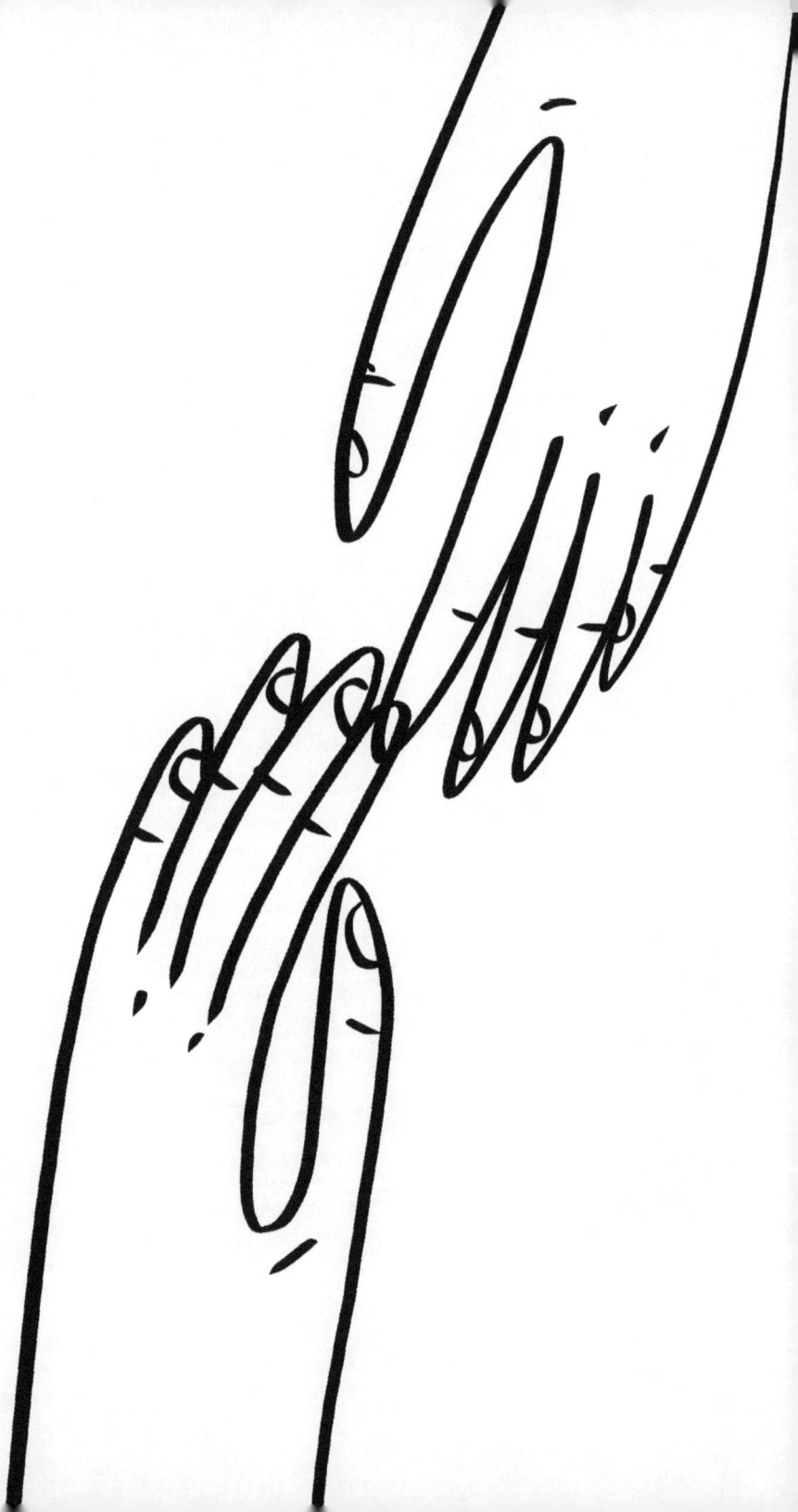

The therapeutic relationship

THE THERAPEUTIC RELATIONSHIP

The therapeutic relationship is one of the most important elements of therapy. People in relationships often talk about their connections with each other, and this is no less important in a therapeutic relationship. If you do not have a connection with your clients, you will not be able to influence them.

Josh McDowell, a Christian author and speaker, explains this well when talking about relationships between parents and children. He suggests that if parents want their children to listen, they must establish some connection to give them a reason to listen. He stated it this way: "Rules without relationships lead to rebellion," meaning if you simply try to tell children what to do without establishing a connection to them, they will rebel. If they have a relationship with their parents, they have something to lose by not following their parents' instructions. The connection and the value a child places on that connection provide the motivation to follow the rules. The child does not want to lose or damage that connection.

The same thing rings true in therapy. If you wish to help someone change or do things differently, you must first establish a connection. Otherwise, they will not last in therapy. They will "try you out," but if the connection is not there they will drop out. Forming this connection or therapeutic relationship is part art, part technique.

HOW TO BUILD A THERAPEUTIC RELATIONSHIP

When I tell new therapists that it's important for a therapist and a client to form a solid therapeutic relationship, I get universal agreement. But when I ask supervision students how to accomplish this, I'm often met with silence or vague strategies such as eye contact, smile, ask questions, open body language, etc. These answers are valid, but they are simply basic conversation and social skills. They're the same skills you would use to teach children with Asperger's how to make friends and listen to the teacher.

Are basic communication skills the only requirement to forming a healthy therapeutic relationship with your client? Is a therapeutic relationship no more complex than a social relationship? I hope that therapists have basic conversation and social skills down before they embark on a career as a therapist! Obviously there is a difference between a simple social relationship and a therapeutic relationship.

Distinguishing between social and therapeutic relationships is important. Social relationships can take forms ranging from simple acquaintance to a friendship. These connections can develop from a variety of sources, including classmates, your child's friends' parents, teammates on a sports team or fellow members of your church. These relationships can be more than acquaintances, but your closest friends fall into a different category of social relationships. Close friends tend to hear more of your thoughts, feelings and struggles. There are some things that you would tell your spouse or a close friend that you definitely would not talk about in casual social relationships.

You may be beginning to see the challenge. As a therapist, what type of relationship do you think is most conducive to therapy—a social, casual one or a close, strong one? A successful therapeutic relationship combines important features of a close relationship (trust, in particular) with strong boundaries, professional insight and a clear focus on purpose and goals. Building a therapeutic relationship as opposed to a regular social relationship takes a special set of skills. Let's look at some of them here:

JOIN THEM

"Meet your client where they are at." We've all heard this advice, but what does that look like? One common mistake of new counselors is they try to solve the problem too quickly or try to reframe the situation. That should not be a first step! Begin by getting stuck with your client. Show empathy. I frequently say things such as "That sucks," "Woah," or "You're kidding, right?" Shedding a tear or handing a tissue can be powerful. Change the tone of your voice and ask questions to indicate that this is difficult or emotional. Pause, and simply show that the situation is overwhelming. Joining them equates to sharing the dilemma. Here's an example of getting stuck with a client.

A woman came into my office seeking counseling for help with her marriage. She showed up alone, as her husband was unwilling to join her. She shared that her husband was an alcoholic, and his condition impacted her and her two children in multiple ways. He caused them financial hardships, racked up some DWIs and even drove drunk at times with the kids in the car. She could never depend on him, and he was unwilling to seek help. She had been in this difficult situation for a couple of years, thought about divorce a few times and even separated, but she never seemed to take that it further. She had been to counseling a couple of times, but nothing ever really changed.

How do you start? Remember, don't start solving ... join. I asked questions about how difficult that must be with someone she loves. We spent time talking about her love for her husband, her heartbreak, and her shattered dreams, and we grieved the loss of her happily-ever-after dream. Pointing out the dilemma a client faces is an excellent way to join them and build a relationship. She was coming in stuck—not stuck in a bad relationship but stuck having to choose between giving up on her dream or hanging on to it.

When clients see that you understand their struggles, the connection is built. Her past counselor (with whom she spent almost two years) spent their therapy time talking about how she should stand up for herself, set better boundaries, be assertive, and not let his behaviors be tolerated. She came in actually saying, "I need help because I never listened to my previous counselor." She clearly had some low self-esteem and shame from that. Interestingly, we worked on all the same things the other counselor was trying to do. The only thing different is we first built a connection by identifying the love she had for her husband and discussing her feeling of being stuck. We frequently had to come back to that theme. The connection we made when she was sharing how she felt stuck was the key to her following through with the goals we set in therapy. She felt understood, believed I knew that her challenges were difficult, and avoided shame because she felt I understood her struggle. Get stuck with your client, and stay a while.

SMALL TALK

Small talk can be awkward and tricky, but you need to engage in some element of conversation with your client outside of therapeutic issues. Life is happening around both therapist and client, and it is necessary to acknowledge and talk about it. Build or strengthen your connection by being human, not a robot focused solely on the dilemma of the hour. Classic small talk about the weather, sports, or current events is essential.

I was terrible at this when I began my career. As a new therapist, my focus was on proving to my client and the world that I knew what I am doing. (I didn't!) I skipped any small talk and just got to work. Clients would come in and sit down, and I would give them a little summary of what we last talked about, what we were working on, and away we would go. Sure, that shows a great work ethic and suggests that I was trying to help my clients get their money's worth, but it did not build a therapeutic connection.

My current approach involves slowing down and using small talk as a means of connecting. It does provide for some interesting moments. I frequently ask a client the typical, "How are you today?" Often I will get some type of answer such as, "I am here, aren't I?" or "Why do you ask that? You know how I am doing," or "What do you want me to say to that?" I tell them, "Well, I am wondering how you are doing, not just how your issue is doing." It often sparks a beneficial conversation about how people are more than their struggles, and they should not let them rule every aspect of their lives. Be careful here, as there are always clients who would love to make small talk all session long. Don't shy away from an awkward transition that sends the message that it is time to get to work, because change is work. I sometimes will simply say, "It is time to get to work."

BOUNDARIES

When engaging in small talk with a client, how do you make it reciprocal? How do you answer questions about your world? If it is small talk time, then it's pretty simple, as small talk never requires disclosure by either client or therapist. Give vague answers about your world, your family, and what you are doing. It is easy to answer in a way that is polite but not revealing. Quickly follow up after your answer to get the topic moving forward.

> Client: "What are you and your family doing this weekend?"

> Me: "One of my kids has a soccer game in Minneapolis." (Give them one more sentence so it reduces the likelihood of a follow-up question, and you are able to give a feeling to help build connection all on your terms.) "We enjoy traveling to different places together." (Now insert a quick follow-up question before they can respond to put it back on them.) "Do you like travel?"

> Client: "Yes; I went to Mexico last year for the first time."

Me: "That sounds great. Would you go again?" *(And we are off to talking about them in Mexico!)*

These little exchanges may not seem important, but they are so valuable. They allow you and your client to connect so your client can see you as a real person. This is vital if you are going to help them with real problems.

Setting boundaries in the middle of a session is difficult, because they will typically involve disclosure. As a therapist, you will learn when the question is being asked as a means of a client trying to find out about you for their purposes or if they are simply looking for instruction. The question could be a way of asking, "Do you know what I am going through?" Fielding a personal question can be jarring, especially when you are new on the job. University textbooks don't teach us how to avoid self-disclosure by shifting focus back on the client to avoid telling too much about you. Some questions are not too difficult and can be handled much like small talk.

Client: "Have you ever had an argument with your wife and you get so mad and say stuff you don't mean?"

Me: "Yep! Many times. It is the worst part about apologizing when you have to say, 'Yeah I only said that to make you mad because I was pretty mad at you.' How do you handle that situation?"

The focus is immediately shifted back to them, and we move on to further the discussion and help the client.

I have had spoken with some therapists who simply respond to that question with, "We are here to talk about you and your wife, not mine." Although that's true and puts up a very clear wall, it also puts the therapist on a whole different level. When you and your client are on different levels, it is hard to have a connection. It is tough to build and keep connections with that answer.

Be aware that the more successful you become at establishing connections, the more likely you will find yourself occasionally fielding probing or intimate questions. Remember, we are only taking about the genuine questions clients are asking that come from a place of gathering relevant information for problem solving. There are a number of times clients ask questions about you that serve no purpose, and you need to keep your guard up and perhaps ignore, deflect, or bypass the inappropriate inquiry.

But what about questions such as, "What would you do if your wife had an affair on you? Would you stay with her?" or, "Would you quit your job if your boss did this?" Pay attention to all the feelings that just occurred when you read those questions. Did you squirm a little? You need to be aware of what just happened, because your body language and your response are extremely important. You can further therapy, or set it back, with your response. What is your response?

You can give the safe boundary-wall answer that you don't talk about your family in sessions, which is politically correct, but think about how that gets interpreted. You essentially just said to your client that you give me all your feelings and I don't give anything back to you! That does not build connection. There is a way to give feelings back and forth but not disclose private intimate feelings that are inappropriate in a therapeutic session with a client.

I see two ways here to answer in a beneficial way that moves therapy along and builds connection. The first response is one you can give if you want to establish limits and erect a strong wall between you and your client. Decline to acknowledge the "your wife" part and simply generalize through your past therapeutic experience.

Client: "What would you do if your wife had an affair on you? Would you stay with her?"

Therapist: "Well you are asking a question that lots of people in this office ask when they are in your situation. I have had experience with people saying they are not staying with their spouse and end up leaving, and I have seen people stay in a marriage after an affair. I have seen outcomes work both positively and negatively both ways. What have you seen with other people?"

And away we go moving on with the discussion.

Remember there is no perfect or even right way to deal with this, but this is how I answered that question.

Client: "What would you do if your wife had an affair on you? Would you stay with her?"

Me: "Wow, I don't really know." *(Said with sadness, because I would be sad if that were true. Show that you are thinking about that scenario.)* "I guess I am not sure. It would be really hard for me to trust her again and move forward. But I also have a lot invested in her and my family, so it would be difficult to throw that all away as well. I am really not sure. Are you leaning a certain way?"

Can you feel the difference in the two responses? Does the first one seem a little cold now? The second response conveys the same message but with more connection and bonding. The answer gives your client safety and encouragement to explore those thoughts. This is just one example of an opportunity to build a therapeutic relationship, and we, as therapists, need to continue to look for these opportunities. A client who feels safe and connected is more likely and willing to do the hard work. I hope you can see that it is possible to share some genuine feelings with your client without blurring boundaries or making it too much about you.

TRANSFERENCE AND COUNTERTRANSFERENCE

I remember first hearing the words transference and countertransference in school and wondering what in the world they meant. They always seemed so cold and foreboding. The way it was taught was that it was a very dangerous thing that you needed to make sure you were aware of at all times. And if you made a mistake, you were doomed—kind of like there is a land mine in the room, so always know where it is and don't ever step on it. Webster's Ninth New Collegiate Dictionary describes transference as:

> *The redirection of feelings and desires and especially of those unconsciously retained from childhood toward a new object (as a psychoanalyst conducting therapy).*

I think a far more understandable definition would be that transference is when a client redirects feelings he has from a situation or person onto a therapist.

The other side of that is countertransference, which is the therapist redirecting his or her feelings from a situation or person onto a client. Now what does that mean and how does it fit into the therapeutic relationship we are trying to build and maintain with our client? Transference and countertransference are quite common and happen often in regular relationships. We often describe this as projection, and we see it in our daily lives and conversations:

"Why are you mad at me? What did I do? You are mad at the kids, not me."

or ...

"Why are you yelling at the kids? What did they do?

"Sorry, I just had a bad day at work."

These everyday occurrences of transference and countertransference are common, but as therapists, we simply need to use these naturally occurring events in a therapeutic manner.

Transference can be awesome. If a client starts to treat you in a way that mimics some of the dysfunctional relationships from his past, you can now work on doing things differently in the session in real time—no more practice, go home, and report back. No more role play! We get to talk about these issues right then and there. This means you will have to point it out the presence of transference and countertransference and be comfortable about talking about how it affects the current situation. If you have that therapeutic relationship, you will be able to do that without your client shutting down.

Pay attention to the themes of how your client talks to you and sees you. You can even seek this out and nurture it by talking about yourself. Here is what I mean: When talking about a client's anxiety, have a conversation about what he thinks of you and how did he handle his anxiety about you? You will hear similarities to how he handles other anxiety-provoking situations.

Did he use any healthy coping skills with you? Why has he kept coming back? How did he get over that anxiety? Ask, "Do you think I am judging you?" or "Why do you think I am not judging you but everyone else is?" These are great ways to look at the transference occurring between the two of you.

Countertransference is trickier and often more difficult to spot. The clear danger in countertransference is therapists putting their issues onto clients. I mentioned this earlier, but it is extremely important to be aware of your own issues. If you know your buttons and triggers, you can see danger coming and steer clear of land mines. If you struggle with certain issues, you need to ascertain whether you able to remain objective and helpful to people with similar issues. Struggling with the same issue as a client can help as far as empathy, but it is sometimes better to focus on a different area of specialization. Those big issues are covered in school, so I want to talk about or the basic, everyday small issues of countertransference. How do you recognize and handle those?

For example, when you see a client on your calendar, sigh, and secretly wish that they would cancel, what is going on there? Why do you feel that way? When answering such questions, be careful not to put all the blame on them and focus on your part in this feeling. This is one of the most beneficial aspects of supervision and staffing cases. As a seasoned therapist, I have been privileged to be in some great staffing situations in which therapists got to bring cases for discussion. Most of the times, the other therapists help by pointing out countertransference issues that I or another therapist did not see.

> **Therapist 1:** "Sounds like you are getting frustrated with your client's reluctance to do any homework."

Therapist 2: "Yes I am. Why is that? Usually it's because I am someone that wants to fix things (hence my job!) and get frustrated when it is not progressing at my rate."

Another example of countertransference frequently shows up in couple counseling. I will sometimes enjoy working with a couple, then notice after a few sessions that the joy is gone. If I pause and identify my feelings, they will typically sound something like, "He is not engaged in the sessions anymore, and she is always negative and shoots everything down." Well if I step back, I realize that I sound like them and have similar frustrations. Success, Tony! You are now in their marriage! Although this is not enjoyable, such a revelation allows you to verbalize feelings towards your client and build that therapist relationship.

It's quite powerful to inform your client of your feelings, share how you don't like feeling that way, and then tell them that you are going to do something a little differently. Saying, "I can't live like that, but you guys may," sends a potent message. I sometimes tell couples, "You guys are going to have to take the lead on how you want the sessions to go, because when I work harder on your marriage than you guys, it makes me want to back off. (Do you think that is a theme they have both experienced at one time or another?)

BE PROFESSIONAL

It is important to convey some type of confidence and assertiveness to convey that you know what you are doing. Show that you have a plan or idea on how to help them feel better or how to help them deal with a theme they are presenting. This is part of the balance that enables you to come across as genuine and understanding. Therapists must balance the need to be empathetic with a client's struggles while conveying that there is hope and an ability to move forward. It is necessary to join them on their journey, but also show leadership that you can help them with their presenting problem.

Being professional also means staying focused on the tenet that it is never about you. Even when you are self-disclosing, it must always be for the purpose of helping the client. As I mentioned earlier, our conversations should have a point and purpose, so stay focused and act in a manner that informs your clients that they are safe and in good hands. How? Act like a professional. Dress like a professional. Maintain a professional looking office and waiting room with organized paperwork and office procedures.

A SPECIAL NOTE ABOUT WORKING WITH KIDS

Kids are a whole different challenge worthy of their own book! But in terms of building a therapeutic relationship, the process takes a lot longer with children. You have to remember that in most situations, children are not seeking help. Instead, someone is making that decision for them. They often don't want to be there.

One of the best ways to begin to build that relationship is to join their world, and that usually involves partaking in playtime. I have played more games of Uno then I care to count! Through the distraction of a game, I can work my way through the methods of small talk, connection, transference, etc. to establish a connection. Be patient working with young children, as the process of building a therapeutic relationship can take significant time. I have worked with a child in which it took weeks to just have them talk to me about behaviors without hiding under my desk! We got there, eventually. He now comes in, sits down, and we do our "work" so we can play.

The key to building all therapeutic relationships is to be real and authentic. If you come across as real, a client will feel invested and work harder to change. Here's another example of what being real looks like: I will often explain what an intervention looks like in therapeutic terms, stating why it is important and the idea behind it. And then I say, "Here is how it will most likely go down in the real world," making the concept feel more authentic and practical.

I will often tell couples stuck in the classic pursuer-distancer circle about the struggle in their relationship and how it shows up in not giving space and chasing the spouse. The best way to get out of this cycle is to have the distancer simply let the pursuer know that they are coming back and they will be able to discuss and resolve the issue after some space. So the homework is to tell your spouse you are coming back when you walk off angry. This makes sense and sounds logical, and it does work. However in the real world, it does not quite go down like that. Giving your client permission to say something more real like, "I will deal with you later!" offers a more authentic look at how it will play out in an actual argument. When you give couples permission to be real, they start to realize that maybe then can do this. And you, in turn, improve the therapeutic relationship you are building with your client.

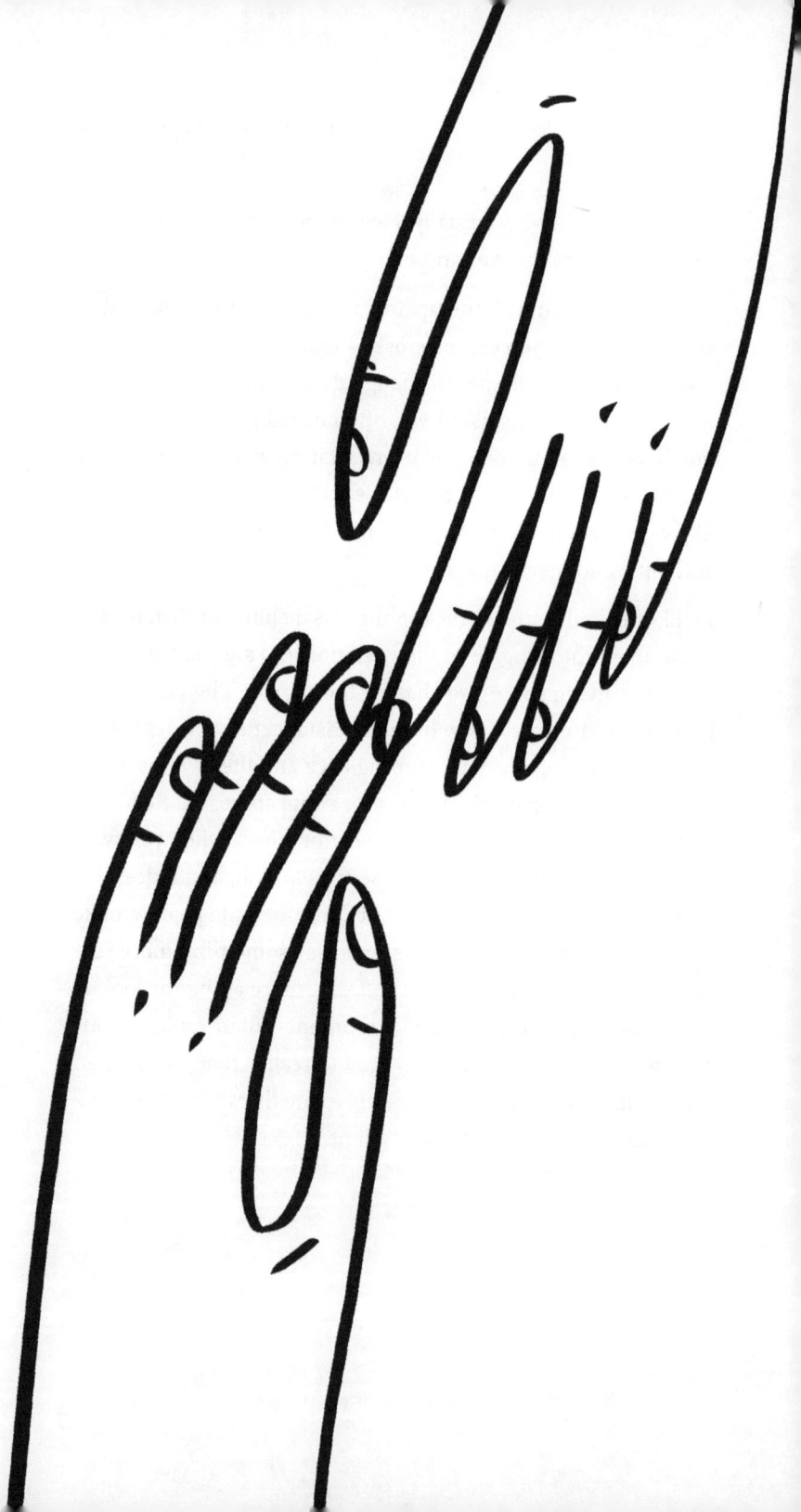

SECTION I: PART IV

The Therapist

THE THERAPIST

When engaged in therapy or providing supervision for others you need to be aware of you and where you are at as an individual. We've discussed the concepts of transference and countertransference, but we need to remember that they are fluid and ever-changing, not just something that comes up and is addressed before moving on. It is essential that you are aware of "where you are at" at all times.

So let's start at the beginning and cover some themes like we did with the client. What motivated you to become a therapist? Why do you want to provide counseling to others? Do you want to make some money? Do you want to have a flexible schedule? Do you want to help others? Did you have a counseling experience that affected you so profoundly that you want to help others? Do you have some issues that you want to work on yourself, so the learning is for you? Are you a therapist simply because someone said you would be good at it? Guess what: All of the answers to the questions above are fine as long as YOU OWN IT! Claim it as yours. What is your theme in providing counseling? You need a theme as well. Why do you do what you do?

What percentage of counselors has attended therapy themselves? A 2004 survey of 800 psychologists conducted by Kenneth Pope and Barbara Tabachnick found that 84 percent had been in therapy themselves.[1] Some counseling programs require students to attend some sessions before graduating. There is no critique or judgement if you have attended therapy; the experience simply provides awareness. What did you learn in therapy how does it affect you today? What if you have never been to therapy, what does that mean? Thinking about these questions allows you to be aware of your issues. We all have them, and we all need to continually deal with them. What are your triggers? Are there any areas or topics with which you would not be helpful as a counselor, or any topics with which you cannot be objective? Do you have soft spots for certain people or issues? Why do you have these? Can you help someone achieve a goal that you don't like or agree with?

If we are trying to teach clients how to make healthy connections with others, we need to start with ourselves.

---

[1] Kenneth S. Pope and Barbara G. Tabachnick, "Therapists as Patients: A National Survey of Psychologists' Experiences, Problems, and Beliefs," Professional Psychology: Research and Practice, 25, no. 3: 247-258.

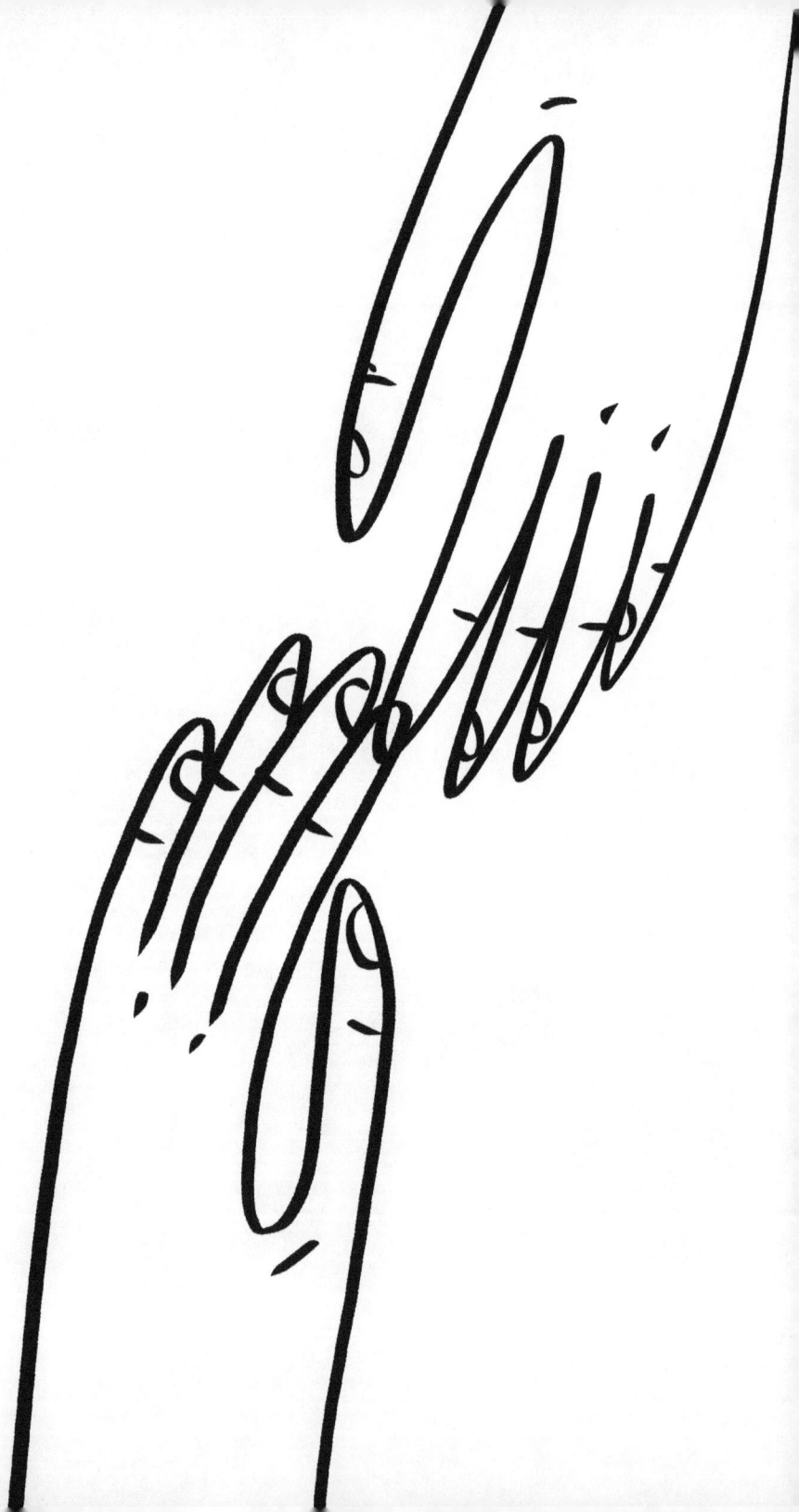

SECTION I: PART V

First Session

FIRST SESSION

Your first session with a client is of utmost importance, as the first impression will be lasting and habits will begin to develop. It is important that you establish good habits from the start. For the sake of discussion here, we'll assume that your client is seeking help on his or her own and is not being forced to come to therapy as part of an agreement involving parole, treatment, etc. Children are an exception, as they frequently do not want to come to therapy and are being asked to come by their parents. Except for a few changes in your method, take a similar approach with kids. I am taking the perspective of a client who is seeking help from a private practice or agency setting.

Therapists face important decisions on establishing an office environment before a patient walks through the door. Some therapists opt for a clinical doctor's-office feel, while others set up a more comfortable living-room feel. Be real and be authentic in what you want it to look like. Several books and articles can assist with your first-time office setup.

We all have our clients fill out paperwork when they reach the reception desk. It's important that we review that paperwork before we meet. Look for clues to help you start to form a picture of who they are. How did they pick you? Where did the referral come from? There are a number of generalities or ideas that you are going to start forming. We can always fine tune and even correct them, so don't worry about if you are getting them right as long as you keep your mind open. You can always adjust later, but you need to get started making the picture.

Let's assume that in reading the paperwork, you learn that the client has been referred from their medical doctor to your practice and you know that doctor fairly well. What can we guess? Well, most likely that they are struggling with some anxiety or depression. Sometimes they will list symptoms such as "sleep issues," "can't relax," etc., but those are some of the basic complaints. This information is helpful as it gives us some idea of what we are getting into. But the most important thing about that information if they are coming from a doctor's referral is this: They are in so much pain, are so uncomfortable, or are so unhappy and seeking change that they went to a doctor to ask for help!

How often do you go to the doctor? Do you go when you are just slightly sick? Do you go when you are mildly irritated with something? When you do go to your doctor, do you tell him all of your stressors? Not likely, and certainly not often. So your client has to be in pretty rough shape if he/she is willing to go in and seek help. Think about the risk they took in seeing the doctor and taking the time to share the struggles of not feeling emotionally/physically well and seeking some relief. The referral doctor may have prescribed some medication, but the client has been referred to you, meaning they have to go through this new-doctor process all over again.

This is who is sitting in your waiting room. You need to remember this picture and those feelings as you approach this first session.

What if the referral comes from a friend of one of your clients? What kind of picture can you begin to create with that? Typically, you can assume that the nature of the issue can be more intimate and personal. What types of struggles do friends share with each other? These are the types of things for which you need to start preparing. How nervous are they now to talk someone who is not a close friend? That is the person sitting in your waiting room.

What if the referral is from a church pastor? What if they came in from an internet or yellow-pages referral? What types of pictures can you start to form from these answers? Who is sitting in the waiting room? These are some of the things that I am looking for when glancing over the paperwork. Did they show up with it all printed and filled out? I have had clients in the past that have showed up 15 minutes early for their appointments and had all the information typed in the blanks! What picture can you make from that? Are they late? Have they asked the receptionist ten questions to ensure they are filling it out right? All of these details help paint a picture.

I've set up my office so that if I am not in a session, I can hear what is going on in the waiting room. It can be extremely enlightening. I have even waited a few extra minutes before seeing people just so I could hear the interactions go on a little longer. Is it a marital couple? Are they arguing? Is it silent? Are they talking? Is it a mom and child? Is the mom yelling at the kid to pay attention? Is he yelling at her? Is he running all over the waiting room? Is he wandering in my office? You can you learn a ton of information in a brief amount of time.

This observation of clients is an old lesson employed by therapists who do home visits. In my early days, I worked as a homebased counselor. Homebased counseling is exactly as it sounds. You go to their house to do therapy. I did not like all the driving around, but one thing that is extremely helpful when you are in their environment is that you can quickly see what is going on in a family. Within five to ten minutes of the start of a home visit, you can often learn the dynamics of a family. It could take five to ten sessions to extract that information in your safe, sterile, office.

Now that we're finally ready to meet our new client, what are some of the little things we can do to begin now to send the message to them. What picture do you want them to have of you? They have started to form a picture of you! These things may seem basic and matter-of-fact, but they are extremely important. Greet them with a smile. Invite them into your office. Don't just walk in. Invite them! I tell them to sit where they want, grab what they want (I have a number of fidgets and toys in my office). Kids will need a little more guidance ("One toy and you must sit on the couch."). I exude a laid-back personality, as I am trying to send that message to them.

Step one is welcome and invite them, and step two is to guide them. Take charge, as they are likely scared and nervous. Your taking some control over the situation will provide some relief. The easiest way to take some control is to tell them what you are going to be doing. Give them an overview of the hour. For a majority of your new clients, this will be their first time in counseling, so they don't know what to expect. I have had clients come into my office and exclaim, "Oh my, you actually have a couch in here! Do I have to lay down on it?!" I reply, "Only if you want to!" I usually give them an overview that goes something like this:

> "Here is what we are going to do today. I am going to explain this paperwork that you signed. I will tell you a little about myself, so you know who in the world you are talking to. I am going to ask you some questions to get a little background information about you. Then, we will see what brings you in today."

This is a way to take control. Share what is going to happen and let them know you have a plan!

I will now walk you through each part of the opening session and my strategy behind the approach.

EXPLAIN THE PAPERWORK

The obvious reason why I am doing this is making sure they understand informed consent. If I am going to try to help them, I want them to know what they are signing up for. I very quickly cover a couple of things, and this exercise typically takes less than five minutes. First, I let them know that everything we talk about is confidential, and inform them of the times when that confidentiality will be broken. (An entire book could be written on the importance of confidentiality.) I typically make sure that kids understand this, as they should be aware of what things I will be telling parents and what things I will not be telling parents.

They next thing I say is that it is their time, their hour, so they should feel free to interrupt me and ask questions. I state, "I want to make sure you get your questions answered." I do this for two reasons. First, I want them to know how long they have and that they need to budget their time. (Some people think that they have the afternoon; others are so scared they feel like it will never end.) To both, I am sending the message that this session has an end. Secondly, I am telling them that they need to be engaged and ask questions. If they are here seeking some help, they are going to have to TELL me what they need help with.

TELL THEM A LITTLE ABOUT YOURSELF

We'll avoid a long discussion on self-disclosure here, but it's important in this initial stage for me to simply tell the client a little about myself. I typically let them know a little about my practice, such as how long I have been practicing and what areas I cover. In my early days, I used to be a little more specific with my resume, as I looked very young and people needed reassurance that I had experience. Unfortunately I do not have that problem anymore! I will tell them a little about myself, based on what I see. If it is a marital couple, I tell them I am married. If it is a family with kids, I let them know I have children. I may tell them that I love to play soccer. I am simply letting them know that I am similar and I want to connect with them.

You cannot connect if you do not share.

I then ask them if they have any questions for me. I will say, "Fair is fair, because I am about to ask them a bunch of questions." Sometimes people will have some questions about experience or where I went to school, but often then are still a little overwhelmed. This provides another way to build connection. Give them some freedom and permission to ask questions, as this is how healthy conversations work.

GATHER SOME HISTORY

It's important to ask the typical questions to gather some personal history, but how deep you dig at the onset will depend on you and your personality. I typically ask just a few basic questions, opting for a strategy that stuff will come out as the sessions unfold. Some clients want to tell you everything that has happened in their lifetimes. I can recall sessions of listening to a 30-year-old client and thinking that they have been talking for 30 minutes and they have not even graduated high school yet! Too much information does not lead to a connection. If you let them talk too much and share too many things, they tend to get overwhelmed. No connection is formed, and those clients tend not to come back. They did not feel as though they made a relationship, or they are too embarrassed by what they said.

You may have to look for ways to find balance in the conversation. Remember how they are feeling and what they are trying to tell you. Can you get the information from other places? Can you request records from other therapists? Some therapists need to have as much information as possible. Some therapists will tell you they don't want past therapists' impressions to cloud their own; they want to form their own insights about the client. Both are valid points, and you'll need to decide your approach. I take the approach of asking the client what they would like me to do. Their answer to this question is often more enlightening then anything in the notes. Do they say, "Yes, please. I want you to know what we talked about. It will be helpful, as then I won't have to go back and explain so much to you." Do they say, "I would prefer that you don't. I never felt as though we got along." Do they say, "No. I don't want my other therapist to know that I am coming here."? All of these answers provide information and give you the opportunity to better know your client.

WHAT BRINGS YOU HERE?

I try to make a clear transition to talking about "the issue," meaning, "What brings you in today?" I often will say, "Those were the easy questions referring to gathering the social history. Now come the hard ones." The first question I ask is, "What brings you here?" I want the client to articulate for what they are seeking help. I will spend a lot more time gathering information and feelings about how they see the struggle. The majority of the session will be this dialogue of them telling me what they see as the problem.

I will ask a number of questions such as:

- "How long has this been going on?"
- "What things have you already tried to fix the problem?"
- "What happened that made you finally call and set up an appointment?"
- "What was the breaking point?"

If it is more than one person in the session, do they have the same view? This needs to be a dialogue and mirror healthy conversations as much as possible.

Clients need to feel some type of hope or relief during the first session. I will frequently tell clients that I am going to be doing at least half of the talking during the first session for a variety of reasons. One, I want to take off some of the pressure. I want to make it feel like a conversation, and I want them to see that we are working together. I also tell them that part of their job/home-work on this first session is to watch me and see what they think of me. I am teaching them about connection right away. We are going to start on a theme of talking about things that they don't normally talk about—the old therapy line of making the covert overt. They are going to be sizing me up, and that's okay.

I want to tell them to size me up and I am going to help them do that! We can even discuss that during the session if they would like. But the first assignment (which I will explain in a moment) is to examine their feelings and see if they feel comfortable with me. I will give them some techniques and ways to do this. I give them an out and say that it is fine if they don't like me. I can help them find someone with whom they feel more comfortable. They need to feel safe, as we are going to working on some tough things. Make it explicit to them that they are looking at the possibility of connecting with you.

You have to give them hope and a plan. At this point, you will not know all of the details of all of their struggles, but you need to be able to offer them some guidance. Let them know that you have had some experience in helping people and you think you can be of some benefit to them. You can share generalities of how you have helped people in the past. but before you do, you need to first know something critical: *What are they hiring you to do?*

Up until this point, we have only been talking about the problem in generalities and gathering information about the problem. Now we need to know clearly what they are hiring you to do.

WHAT ARE THEY HIRING YOU TO DO?

This is the most important question to ask, and you will likely find yourself reminding them of their answer many times during future sessions. We may even have to change from time what we are working on. The importance of this question is that it helps create a realistic honest answer of what they are working on. The initial question often stumps people, yielding an answer of, "I don't know." If we as therapists accept this answer, we will likely fail. We have to first figure this out.

Many therapists never get to this point. They hear a number of symptoms, form a treatment plan, and start working. The client will come for a few sessions, participate, and perhaps feel like things are working, but usually after about two-to-three months, they will drop out. Why?

Ask a client who had this experience with another counselor when you are doing your history discussion. If they say they have been to counseling before, ask them about what they learned and what were they trying to fix? You will hear things like, "I didn't learn anything. We talked and he was nice, but we never really got anywhere. He just listened." Those are clear signs that the therapist never clarified the problem. I get frustrated when I ask someone who has been in counseling in the past, "What did they work on or learn?" and they say, "I don't really know." That is a counselor problem not a client problem. If they say, "I did not want to work on things or was not serious about working on the problem, that is likely on the client. But it is the therapist's responsibility to clarify with them what they are hiring you to do.

Sometimes, a client will explain what they are hiring you to do, and you need to ask for clarification or ask, "Is that what you are *really* wanting? And most importantly: *Do you want that job?* Sometimes, with the jobs that clients first explain to me, I must tell them I do not want the job or cannot help them with the issue. For example, a man may come in and his answer to the question of "What are you hiring me to do?" is something like this:

Man: "My wife says that I have an anger problem, and if I don't stop getting angry she is going to leave me. You need to help me so I don't get angry."

Me: "I don't want that job. I don't think I can do that. I can't help people stop getting angry."

Man: "Well that sucks." (I love guys like this—honest and real!)

Me: "So is your wife telling you that you cannot or are not allowed to get mad anymore, or she will leave you?" (Reframe, and make it clear what he feels is different than what is being asked.)

Man: "No. I guess not. Everyone is going to mad, right? She just does not like how loud I get and how much I yell."

Me: "I will take that job. If you are hiring me to help you not yell as much when you get mad, I think I can help."

This is simple little exchange that is powerful and builds a therapeutic alliance. We are now focused on something realistic, and the client is validated that he can be mad and angry. We are working on managing his anger, not eliminating it. That is also an important distinction that the man may need to make to his wife.

Look at the examples below, and compare them to the rephrased problems:

Do you want these jobs as a therapist?

"Make my son listen better."

"Make my daughter stop cutting."

"Save my marriage."

"Help me to stop worrying so much."

"Help me not be so depressed."

Or would you rather have these jobs?

"Help my son follow directions more often."

"Help my daughter feel safe, secure, and confident."

"Figure out why I am not connecting with my spouse."

"Help me figure out why I can't relax and trust myself."

"Help me figure out why I don't feel as though I am okay."

The second set of jobs are ones you might want, and you want your client to know that is why they are here. I will frequently remind people as our sessions go forward about what we are working on. With kids, I make them repeat it almost every session. (I have them repeat the goal that the kid, the parent, and I came up with). It's extremely important to nail down exactly what a couple is hiring me to do when conducting marital therapy, as each member of the couple is often not hiring you to do the same thing!

If you can agree on a job, then you also need to make sure you paint a picture that it is going to take hard work, as we are changing the way a client has approached and tried to solve the problem in the past.

HOMEWORK ON THE FIRST SESSION

I typically end the each client's first session with this statement:

"When you go home I want you to talk about me!"

I then go on to explain.

"We are going to be working on identifying and sharing feelings and how they affect your actions." *(I'm a cognitive behaviorist at heart!)* "So I want you to be able to share what you think of me. I am not going to ask you what you think. I don't think I want to know! I want you to share what you think about me and what you think about coming here with your spouse (or child or friend). If you tell your spouse, 'Tony had a messy desk and toys all over his office and wore a blue shirt,' what has your spouse learned? Nothing! But if you say things like, 'That is the smartest guy I have ever talked to,' or 'He is the dumbest guy I have ever met,' now we are getting somewhere. The goal at the end of the homework is for your spouse to be able to verbalize how you feel about me and how you feel about being here. It is a safe subject to start the lessons of facts vs. feelings. Your feelings are not wrong, and you need to communicate them in a way that gets heard."

This works with marriage clients, parents with kids, and even individual clients. I will have an individual client share it with a close person or even have the client talk out loud to themselves about their feelings. A couple of other instructions need to be given. It is important that you start to change and break patterns, so you need to ask couples, "Who talks the most?" and, "Who shares the most feelings?" Typically, it will be the female, unless there is a dominant man who will talk a lot but not share feelings. In general, you want the person who uses the most words to go *last*. If it is a kid, they need to go first. Otherwise, Mom will typically do all the talking, and everyone else will go, "Yes. I agree with what she said."

This type of response can be a problem in couples therapy, because if a woman who felt as though she just bared her soul is met with her husband simply agreeing, she might feel as though she is not connected with him, he is not invested, and he does not care. He, however, might have just had her take all of his thoughts about me and generally does not have anything to add. If you reverse the order of speaking, he will have to share something, she will feel connected, and she will still have plenty to add. It's similar with kids, as they often feel as though their feelings don't matter or their feelings are wrong. I want them to know that we are going to be sharing feelings, and I want them all agreeing on what they are hiring me to do.

I usually end the first session by telling the clients do the assignment, talk about therapy, and then call back if they want to get started on what we talked about. I do not try to get them to set an appointment up right away (I admit this is probably not the best business strategy) but I want them to go home and think about the session. I often use a little more self-disclosure right at the end to continue to build the connection by saying, "I don't like to feel pressured to do things, so I don't want others to feel that was as well." Some follow that advice and go home, and some ignore my advice and schedule an appointment right away.

This is how I conduct my initial sessions, and I hope that you can tailor some of these methods to fit your needs and style. You many not feel comfortable in doing some of these things, and that is fine. A majority of the therapists I know have their first sessions last an hour-and-a-half, but I choose to squeeze everything within an hour. My belief is that more stuff will come out during subsequent sessions, and the first session should focus solely on about getting a handle on the problem and establishing a connection with the client.

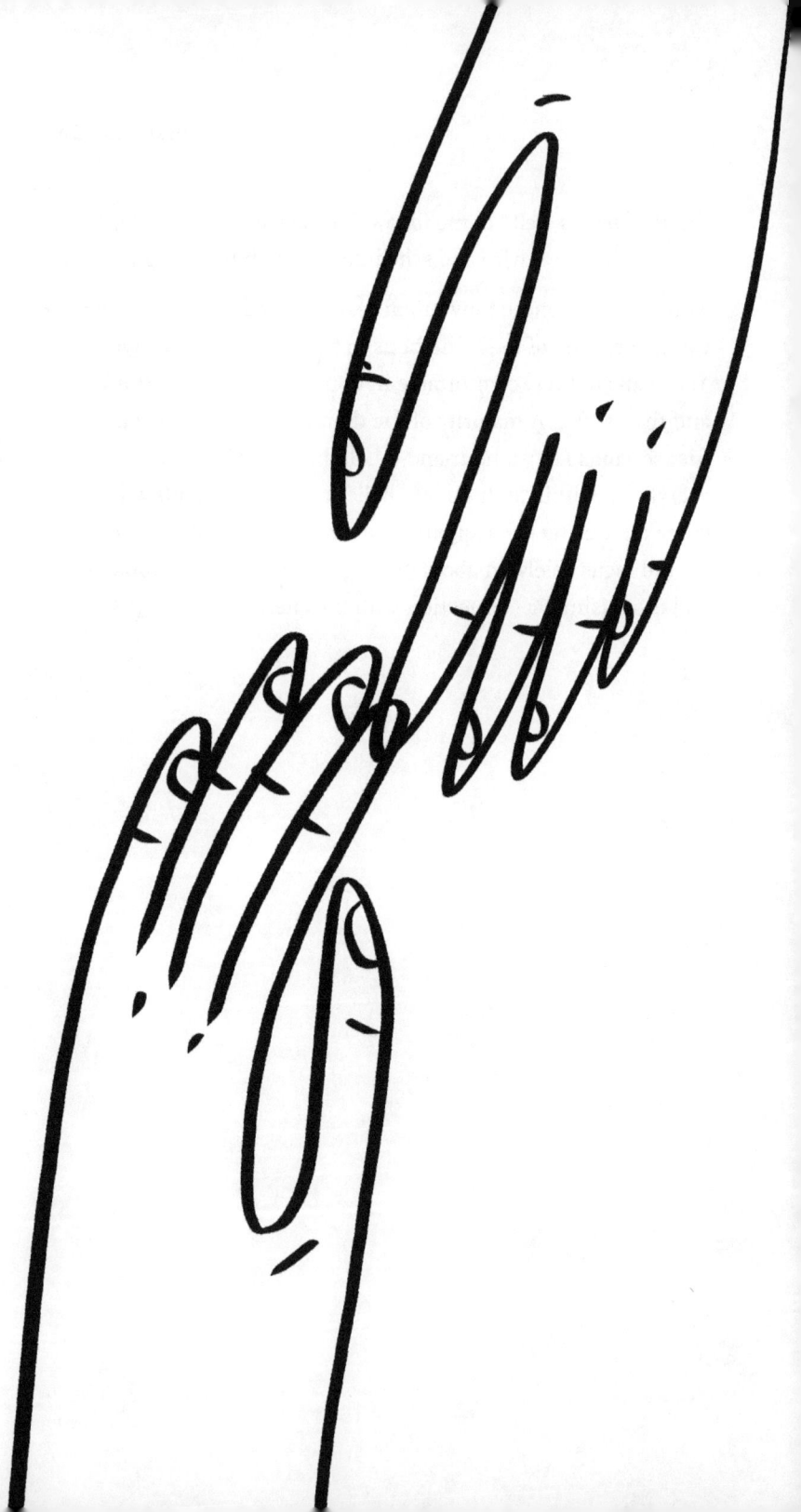

Treatment plan

TREATMENT PLAN

With the first session complete, it is now paperwork time.

The dreaded treatment plan can be difficult and overwhelming, but it's an important document for therapists, clients, insurance companies, agencies, etc. Therapists typically need to write a treatment plan fairly quickly after meeting a client, and it's commonly required after the first session. That's no easy task after just one session, so such a plan will not be very specific, opting for generalities that hit the main presenting problem. I tend to keep things general in written records, anyway, but treatment plans evolve over time. Focus the plan on the main goal of what they are hiring you to do. You will have to write that in therapeutic terms, but that premise should be at the core of all of your interactions.

What is the theme on which you are working? For example, if the agreed upon goal is, "Help me learn how to do a better job parenting my child," the treatment plan in more therapeutic terms would read something like, "Develop and implement positive coping skills in parenting." This statement encompasses the main theme, and you can always work on objectives and smaller goals that reflect or refer back to the main theme. The smaller goals may be to teach coping skills, so educate clients on whatever behavioral issues the child may have. Avoid negatively framed goals by cognitively reframing negative behaviors to look at them from a different view. For example, instead of declaring a treatment to stop yelling at the kids, write it as "Implement healthy boundaries." These objectives or smaller goals are all based on the original goal or theme. When writing the treatment plan, think about how to make this theme work better for them. Where are they getting stuck, and do they need more skills to do things differently?

The treatment plan is what you put down on paper, but there is different part of forming a treatment plan that depends on connection. What are you going to do in the session to help them? What is your plan for helping them change their theme or help them develop a healthier theme? *You must have a plan on how you are going to help someone change.* There are many different ways and a variety of different theories to get to where you want to be. This is one the hard parts of supervision, especially when you are staffing a case or working in collaboration with other therapists. They will ask, "What is the right way to address this?" There is not *a* right way; there are many. As long as you have the goal and the problem clearly defined, there are many techniques and theories to address the problem.

When therapists lack a treatment plan, they will sometimes make a declaration such as "I think I know what is wrong." The problem is they don't have a clear idea on what to do next.

Any theory or approach can work, but if there's no identification of a theme and a treatment plan built around that theme, a client can lead *you*, typically in circles. You need to lead them. Remember, they hired you. They told you the problem and then asked you to address it, not simply talk about it or continually look at it from different angels. When you know the theme and identify the problem, you will start to see it show up in a multitude of situations. It will provide numerous times to practice and do things differently.

HOMEWORK (ONGOING)

My twofold purpose in assigning homework is to gauge how serious the client is about change and to give them specific ways to do things differently. It's easy to get an answer on the first purpose if a client continually blows off the assignments, saying things such as, "It will never work." You need to go back to the original question, "What did you hire me to help you with?" When a client continues to come in without trying your suggestions, he or she is telling you: "I am hiring you to keep me the same!" (This actually happens a lot.) I tell those clients, "You can do that for free, and you don't need my help." We may need to change our job description. Often, you can clarify the situation with some healthy reframes of what they are telling. (Here's my cognitive approach showing up again.)

Let's pause for a quick review from what you learned in school about reframing. A reframe is simply taking what the client is telling you and saying it in a different way to illustrate how it sounds. These can be powerful, and I use them frequently. Often, simply saying the consequences or result of what they think, thus taking their thoughts to a logical conclusion, is a powerful way to show how their thinking is flawed.

For example, when I was working with a client on her frustration about her husband's poor listening skills, his lack of helping around the house with the children, and his lack of affection toward her, we developed the theme of her wanting to feel more valuable and loved. It's a strong yet reasonable general theme that that avoids making her feel as though there is something wrong with her. I assigned a variety of the homework that taught her how to share these issues with her husband. I asked her to be clear and real with her feelings instead of simply sharing her frustrations or times in which he let her down

She continued to come back and say how her husband is still not doing what he is supposed to do. I would ask her if she told him how she felt in the way we practiced. She would always have a reason for why she did not try it. So I did a reframe and asked if she really wanted things to be different, as I was thinking based on her actions that she was hiring me to help her just accept how things were. I reframed this *accept* goal clearly to her by saying something along the lines of, "I think maybe we should work on accepting that this is how your husband is going to be. He is not going to help you out around the house and not going to help with the children, and you are going to be feeling left out. But if we can help you come to acceptance of this and not have it bother you so much, I think you would feel better and not get so upset when it happens." Typically she will look at me and say "That really sucks! I don't want that!" and we come back to, "Well, I have an idea or how to address this and we come back to the original homework with a renewed sense of focus.

This brings up the second issue with homework: it needs to be difficult. Why did the woman in the above example not share how she felt? Why was she unwilling to do things differently? Because it is hard to share feelings. It is easy to share, "I am mad, because you did not help clean the kitchen." It is hard to say, "I felt abandoned yesterday." Homework needs to be uncomfortable! Growth results from pain. We all understand growing pains from our teen years in dealing with a leg that hurts or soreness in our adult years in returning to exercise or typing on a keyboard for the first time in a while. (I am dictating my next book!) The same is true with emotional growth—it results from doing new and difficult things. I did not tell my client to go home and yell a little louder at her husband when he was not helping her. That would be easy for her to do, and she has already done that approach many times. I tell clients all the time that if I give you a homework assignment and you excitedly say, "I can do that," then I just gave you the wrong assignment. If I tell you your homework assignment and you say, "I don't know if I can do that," I got it right.

The homework should be difficult to complete, but the instructions should be simple. In the above example, the homework assignment was, "Tell your husband how you feel." That is a simple sentence that can be remembered and repeated. That is what you want for homework. Don't make the assignment seem too big and complicated. Convey that it can be done in the real world and in real time. Just because the instructions are simple doesn't mean that the assignment is easy. "Run a marathon." That is a simple assignment, but to complete the marathon you need to train, eat right, and show dedication to see results. An assignment of, "Say how you feel" will take the same tenacity and approach. Don't get caught up in giving big complicated homework assignments, and resist the urge to give them a bulk of assignments.

This is, again, where the personality of the therapist shows up. I am not one to give lengthy workbook and reading assignments. Sometimes I will have clients ask me to give them this type of homework, and I may oblige with some supplementary assignments, but these will not replace those that address our main goal. Here's another example of the theme of being in a relationship with your client. It is easy to give homework, but you can quickly fall into the role of teacher. Although we certainly will provide education to our clients, that is not our sole purpose. If we are in a relationship with our client, it is easy to confront challenge and give them assignments that are beneficial and impactful.

Finally, take time to reflect and organize your approach. This is especially important when starting out, and it's one of the most valuable aspects when staffing cases or performing supervision. It's extremely helpful to take a moment to gather your thoughts and consider how to present your case and state the identified themes and the direction you are headed. Although you can't staff every case after ever session, you can do this in a small way when you write your notes. Keep your notes simple and basic to protect what is said in session, but be sure to keep in mind the client's themes and plans. The work can lead to a more beneficial next session, as it provides time to reflect and edit the plan.

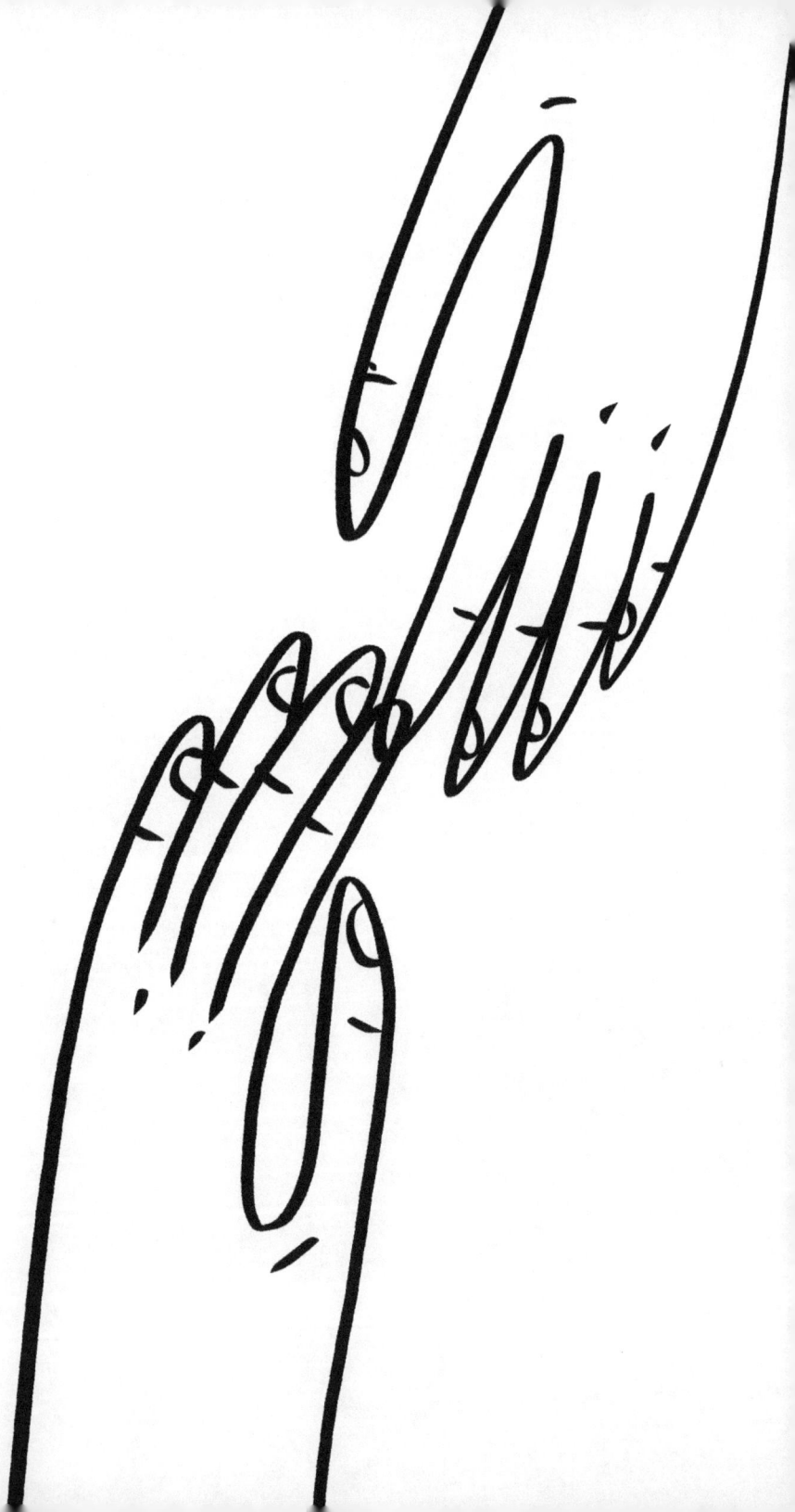

Universal Themes

UNIVERSAL THEMES

It takes practice and experience to think of people's issues in terms of themes, as it's easy to get lost in the little problems that people bring forth. You need to ensure that clients tell you enough about their problems and issues to get a good handle on what is happening, but you don't want to let them stray too far. This is especially important early on, as they may get overwhelmed and feel as if they shared too much. A client who feels embarrassed and exposed will likely not return.

Some seasoned therapists call this "emotional vomit." A client will come in and just unload everything! Although it can be healthy to let such things out, if the purge lacks context or balance it can result in a client feeling only temporary relief mixed in with some shame about how much they have exposed. It is your job to balance what they give you and how fast they give it to you. You may need to use phrases such as, "That sounds as though that had quite an impact on you. We may need to go and explore that more in a later session. Tell me what other factors bring you in today." The transitions may feel clunky, but you need to make sure you show some leadership in how the session goes while still getting the information that you need.

DON'T GET LOST IN THE DETAILS

To remain open to identifying themes, step back and don't get lost in the details. I can recall times when I am telling a therapist about a client (no names are ever given) and noting that I am stuck, and they will ask me questions about the person that are not relevant to the discussion. I will ask them why are they asking that question. Am I missing something? Then they say, "I don't know I was just curious." Curiosity often leads you down wrong path.

As an example of this, I remember staffing a case about an individual who was struggling with self-worth issues due to some difficult things in their past. I said something along the lines of, "I have this client with whom I am having trouble getting to open up about their feelings. She works in a bank and does a great job with people, but will occasionally have some struggles with her coworkers. She can't seem to identify or see that she does a good job herself." Another therapist who was listening to me staff the case then asks, "What bank does she work at? My friend works at a bank. I wonder if it is the same one. She has difficulty with some of the peers at her bank as well." This is a great example of getting lost in details.

You will recognize these types of details often in the first session in which people try to give you the story of what is going on, but they insist on starting the story from the beginning. The client will feel the need to tell you her mother's life story and retell how her mother was raised in order to explain why her mom said something hurtful and your client did not know how to handle it. If you are not careful, you can spend your time validating and offering deeper insights into why her mother acts the way that she does. These are all helpful things and maybe something to cover later in counseling, but not in that moment. In that moment, you have to stay focused and see the big picture of *why* was she telling you that story and what was your question that sparked that story. Did your client answer the initial question? What is the theme of what she said? Are you learning that she has trouble expressing her feelings or setting boundaries? Have you already heard a similar story about how her husband hurts her and or treats her? How about her job? Does she tell you a story of feeling taken advantage of at work and having to do everything because no one else will? Can you see the theme? Does your new client need help with setting boundaries? Getting caught up in the details of your client's stories can result in you getting lost and missing the theme.

DON'T PROBLEM SOLVE

Another tendency to avoid is jumping too quickly into problem solving. It may seem perfectly logical that our purpose is to hear our clients' issues and offer suggestions on how to handle them. It sounds like a good idea, especially when you are a new therapist fighting that urge in your head saying, "I have got to give them something they are paying me to help them!" Jumping in on problem solving the first problem a client shares stops that person from giving your more information. You may provide some temporary relief, but you also setting up a pattern for how counseling will work. They share a problem, and you offer suggestions. They share another problem, and you offer more suggestions. This is a frequent mistake of new therapists, keeping clients coming in for a while but never addressing the core issues. Clients often will drop out, as they will feel as though counseling never really helped. If you feel the need to "give them something," share generalities of how you may help them, but let them know that right now you are just gathering information to find out what they are wanting.

THE ONE BIG THEME

In the next section, we will address common themes, but there is a fundamental theme that is present in all of us: *We all have the need to feel accepted and feel as though we fit in.*

It can be verbalized in different ways, and you can call it feeling loved and valued or identifying your purpose, but it revolves around the concept of acceptance and belonging. I like to keep it simple and express this theme as the belief that "YOU ARE OKAY. You are loved, valued, and accepted.

Unfortunately, a lot of people do not feel this way. This grounding and sense of peace that you are loved and okay is an essential part of the human experience. When you feel loved, accepted, and valued, or know that you are okay, you have a framework for approaching and handling life that helps you combat and overcome its challenges. It also allows you to be present for others, and by being present you continue to feel loved and valued.

This is a universal concept, but my personal perspective here is rooted in my belief that the best way for someone to truly feel love and acceptance is through Jesus Christ. He is the ultimate person who has said that you are okay and just fine. You may not feel it yet, but Christ has said, "I love you just how you are. You are okay. In fact, you are so okay that I am willing to die for you!"

This feeling allows you to move forward with how to approach life and how to address others. If you want to get technical, this is at the basis of almost all of the struggles that draw people to counseling. Knowing that you are okay, believing you are okay, and acting in such a way is the remedy for a majority of the struggles we face. The challenge is to learn how to believe it or feel it and act that way, and that's where therapy comes in. When you help people identify and feel this acceptance, you have helped them take a tremendous leap toward being more successful in life—and by success I mean feeling at peace and living a satisfying life. It's important that we as therapists always keep this underlying theme in mind when looking at the variety of ways people try to fix the feeling of not being okay. As we go forward and look at specific themes of how people act, they all draw from a framework of trying to feel better and fix something that makes them feel not okay, not loved, or not valued. Keep this in mind as we look at specific themes.

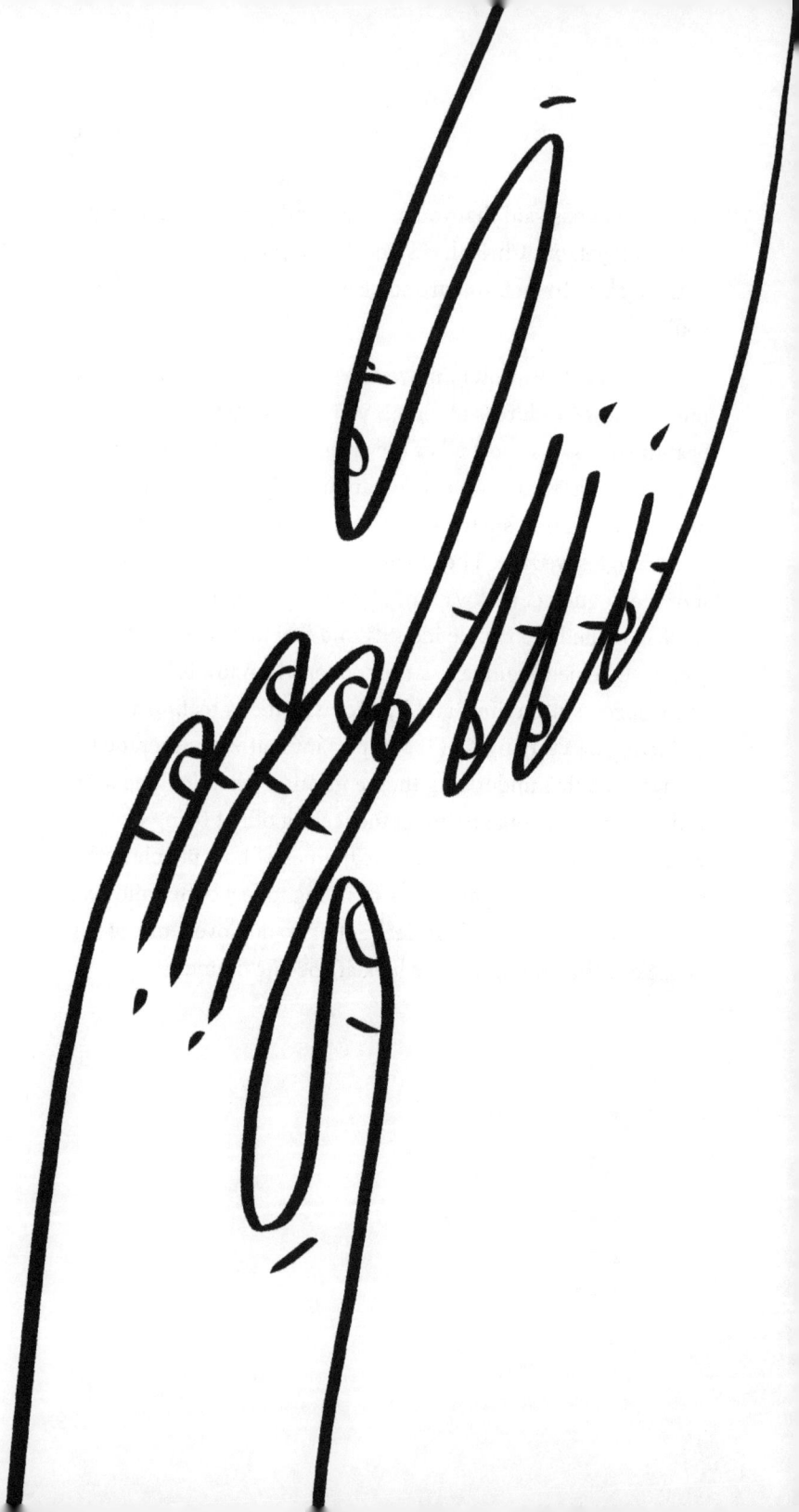

SECTION I: PART VIII

Individual Themes

INDIVIDUAL THEMES

I just covered the theme that tends to be present with everyone—*We all have the need to feel accepted and feel as though we fit
in.* We are now going to look at some individual themes. These
are not diagnoses, per se. They're just general common themes
that I have seen in therapy. They do not mean there is something "wrong" with a person. They're just indicative of a certain
way a person sees the world and how that way may be causing
some issues. These themes provide ways to help clients work in
generalities and improve how they feel, instead of working on a
topic or issue at a time. Let's look a few common themes you'll
likely come across in counseling others.

THEME: YOU ARE RESPONSIBLE FOR OTHER PEOPLE'S FEELINGS

One common theme seen by therapists is when clients feel as
though they are responsible for other people's feelings. This
can show up in clients who are consistently worried about how

other people will feel or respond if they say "no." Clients will also talk about how they fear how people will feel if they cause any type of discomfort for them. Sometimes, parents will feel as though they are responsible for their children's feelings and become overprotective. I have seen some parents go as far as doing all their homework for their children, as the parents didn't want them to feel bad if they would fail an assignment! This responsibility for other people's feelings or happiness can grow so out of control that it has been given its own term— codependency. It is interesting that if you look up codependency on the internet, you will find a variety of information, but it's absent from the DSM 5 (Diagnostic and Statistical Manual of mental disorders 5th edition), the book that labels and explains mental health disorders. Some say that codependency is a collection of symptoms so it is labeled as a syndrome, while others say it is a legitimate disorder. It has also been labeled as dependent personality disorder.

Regardless of how it's classified, we as therapists need to recognize the theme of codependency when it surfaces. How do we help people who are struggling with it? Can we convey to our clients how this worrying about how others feel impacts their life in a negative manner? Can we help our clients see that if they consistently put themselves last, they enable poor behaviors in the people around them and create even more difficulty in their life? By approaching this as a theme, it allows us to have more interventions and address the issues in a deeper manner. How does an individual who has this theme of feeling responsible for others feel? Sad? Overwhelmed? Frustrated? Is this why they came into therapy? Too often, they will come in saying their issues are about how they need to do better because they are failing or that their life is not going well, when in reality they might not need to do better but need to do less.

A mom who comes in stating that she is frustrated and depressed because her son is struggling in school and not taking his schoolwork seriously might ask for ideas on how she can be a better parent to help her son show more initiative. Notice how much ownership she is taking in the problem and how little she is giving to him! She is coming to therapy, not him!?! If you as a therapist simply tell her to set better boundaries and make her son do his homework and not do it for him, he will have to take more ownership of it. But that will only happen when *he* feels the pressure, not his mom. It's a rather easy answer and makes sense.

I have even had therapists I am supervising come up with a basic behavioral plan on how to have the son sit down and do his homework. If this is all you do, you may make a little progress on her acting more firmly with her son. But I am not sure that it will last, and even if it does, the troubles with her son will most likely switch to something else. Mom will try a few times to be firm, make a little progress, and then drop out of therapy. Why? We did not help her change her theme; we addressed it only on the surface of how the theme shows itself. If you spend a little more time exploring how often she makes a choice to be responsible for other people's feelings, she will see the expanse of how often this happens and the expense of its impacts and costs. Watch for other things as she tells you about the homework problem, making comments about other things such as:

> "Well he was mad and wanted to play with his friends who were knocking at the door, so I had to let him go. They were wanting to play with him and I needed to go help my daugh-

ter with her piano lessons and get supper going before my husband got home. So I just let him go. And by the time he came back it was suppertime and getting late, so I just gave him the answers and had him write them down, else he would be crabby the next day."

If we walk with her through that statement and point out to her the number of times that she makes choices so that other people do not have to suffer, we will show how she is enabling her family to continue this dysfunctional pattern and give our client a deeper understanding of what is going on. We are helping her set healthy boundaries and allow others to have some uncomfortable feelings. This is much better than helping her do better with her son and his homework. Our goal is to help her see this as a lifestyle that will make her feel better. Clients tend to stay in counseling and improve when they see the importance and how a theme impacts their life. If you can get them to start looking for the theme, that is the first step toward change! I hope you are beginning to see the power in identifying how themes work in people's lives.

THEME: YOU ARE NO GOOD

Another theme that you will frequently identify is one in which the client struggles with self-esteem/low confidence/low self-worth. This can take on a lot of different names, but it's important that a client recognize this theme in their own struggles. I often let clients name it for themselves, and then we go with whatever name they provide as our theme. Listen for this theme in your client's struggles. It will show up over and over again. Helping a client identify how often a particularly theme shows up is often powerful and enlightening. With the theme of low self-confidence, clients will be reluctant to try different coping skills or techniques out of fear that things will not work out. Or they may self-sabotage by saying things such as, "I can't do that" or, "I will try, but it I never seem to do things right." Can you help the client see that this type of low confidence affects not only the problem that they are coming in for but other areas of their life as well? Ask questions to help clarify their understanding:

- "Do you have those feelings at work?"
- "With your husband?"
- "How do others respond when you are displaying this lack of confidence?"
- "Do people cheer you on or withdrawal and avoid you when talk in a self-defeated manner?"
- "Do your children notice that or do you hide it from them?"
- "Are you teaching them to doubt and second guess themselves?"

You most likely will have to go slowly and give them time to think and process all of these questions. You do not need to tackle all these questions in one setting. It is often helpful to have the client reflect and see how this belief impacts not only themselves in more ways than they originally thought, but also those close to the client. By establishing the theme they are working under, they will be more motivated and engaged to change it.

THEME: MUST DO IT RIGHT / PERFECTIONISM

This theme is usually easy to identify, as often the client is aware that this is a theme in their life and it might be the reason why they are seeking help in therapy. It will not take much work to point out the existence of the theme, but clients some-

times miss how perfectionism shows up in feelings and relationships. They will see how it causes stress in their life with
things, but miss how it causes stress with people. This theme
of having to do things "right" can be seen in a variety of anxiety
disorders. Clients who struggle with Obsessive Compulsive
Disorder (OCD) will often be able to identify that they need to
work on breaking some of their dysfunctional patterns such as
hand washing or cleaning. They can tell you they "know" they
don't need to do the compulsion and that it is impacting their
daily life, but they will often have limited insight into how this
behavior may impact those around them. Clients have even less
insight on the theme of needing to *feel* right. They are not aware
that the compulsion to *do* right is easier to see than the compulsion to act and *feel* a right way, which can be just as powerful
but more difficult to identify.

If you listen to what your client is saying, you will start to hear
them talk using words such as "have to," "must," or "need to."
Not only might you notice that they using these words often,
you will start to identify the situations in which these words
come up frequently and connect them to stress or challenge in
their life. Further exploration of these sentences will help the
client identify that this rigid drive to do things correct shows up
not just in cleaning and hand washing, but in how they view the
world. This need to do things correctly might be causing more
stress in more areas than they are aware. And when they are
under more stress, what do they do to cope? You guessed it—by
trying to control things and do things right. If they can't feel
right at least they can do right! This increasing compulsion to
do things right is an effort to "forget" or distract from the feelings that they are having, which are often accurate and healthy.

Just because a feeling does not feel good, does not mean it is not healthy. If this theme of being a perfectionist causes them to make rules not beneficial to them, then our goal is to help them change the rules. They made the rules that are causing them stress, so they can change them.

I often hear clients come in staying that they have this way of living their lives and they express the expectations put have of themselves. They express frustration that they can't meet their expectations and ask for help to meet them. I tell them, "Well, I am pretty sure you have tried pretty hard to meet them and have exhausted a long list of approaches. How about instead of trying harder to follow these expectations, we change the expectations?" An example:

Client: "I am so overwhelmed. I have to get the house cleaned before our friends come over on Saturday night for supper."

Therapist: "How long will it take you to clean the house?"

Client: "It usually takes me about 4-5 hours a week, but I need to wash the windows since they need be done as well."

Therapist: "Can you tell me why the windows need to be done before your friends come over for supper?"

Client: "Well I need to have a clean house before company comes over!"

Therapist: "Where do the windows fit in?"

Client: "Well you can't have someone over to house if your house is not clean, and my widows are not clean from winter. If my house is not clean, it is a poor reflection on me and how I run my house and family."

Therapist: "Who told you that?"

Client: "I don't know. I guess it would be my mom. She always had a clean house. She said that people will judge you on how your house looks."

Therapist: "What do you think of that?"

This provides an opportunity to explore the rules passed on by her mom and examine if she has (or should have) the same ones. Often upon discussion, the client will be able to identify that her mother did not work outside the home and had a lot of time to clean the house. She will also be able to identify that just because mom had that view that a clean house is a reflection on your success doesn't mean that she needs to hold to that rule. She will see that she works outside of the home and judges her success by a variety of ways, from success at work to being a supportive wife, to being a good mother AND all of her mother rules. Helping her change her theme of "must do it right" to "What do you must do right and what don't you have to be perfect on?" can provide a new perspective that helps the client begin to change her theme.

Sometimes a client will say, "But I feel better when I have a clean house." Then we need to explore what they said earlier when they were overwhelmed. They don't *have to* clean the house; they *want to* clean the house. Embracing and accepting that will also reduce the stress. Instead of framing it as, "I need to get this done," you help the client see it as, "I enjoy cleaning, as it makes me feel good." There's nothing wrong with that statement, as it takes away the need and the judgment and puts it into a more healthy perspective. The client will just need to get used to saying it to herself as a reminder.

THEME: I WON'T LET OTHERS TAKE CARE OF ME / TRUST

This theme is not as easy to identify as some of the others, as it often sits subtly under the surface. This is usually identified in clients who upon looking at their history start to identify that they have made some choices in situations that don't make sense. They don't usually come seeking help by saying, "I need help trusting people." What brings them in is often a cover of the real problem.

Clients with this theme tend to begin therapy with problems such as, "My husband says that I am distant and hard to reach, but he is really needy." This is obviously a theme that is present with a number of adoption and attachment issues—situations in which people make life harder by pulling away from others instead of asking for help. It's a hard theme to identify, as often the client will explain it away it terms of their not needing help or expressing that those around them would never help anyways. "No one ever helped me before. Why would they do that?"

When talking, you begin to hear that they never asked for help in a certain situations. Dig a little deeper and you may find that they never ask for help. Interestingly, they are often extremely willing to offer help to others. You will begin to hear things such as, "I don't get along very well with others," or, "I am often accused by husband of not caring." When you are able to identify this theme, you will start to hear it show up everywhere in their life. This can be a difficult theme to change, as a client may have learned this at a very young age and have very good reasons for not trusting others or not asking for help. This theme is usually triggered by past hurt. The best strategy to tackle this theme is to help your client see it as past hurt and identify ways to begin to trust slowly.

THEME: I AM NO GOOD / DAMAGED

This is a theme that is also typically hidden from others. Clients who have this theme may express that they are struggling in life because they are no good or are simply destined to struggle. Unfortunately, there is often some type of abuse that the client has experienced. Clients can make sometimes the connection between how they were treated and how they see the world, but sometimes they cannot.

If you listen to a client struggling with this scenario talk long enough about whatever brought them in, you'll begin to hear hints that they approach situations from a manner in which they believe that they are not worthy to have options or thoughts, or they don't speak up on when they feel taken advantage of. If I ask if they have ever been in abusive situations as a young child, often I will hear, "Yes, but that it was a long time ago. What does that have to do with anything?" They say, "I am over that." Well the client may think they are over that incident, but I am not sure they are over the theme of, "You are no good."

It can be therapeutic to walk with a client through the things they have learned and taken away from abuse, oftentimes things of which they were not even aware. I will frequently listen for anything that is negative, self-defeating, or sounds as though they don't believe they matter. Then I will say, "That sounds like the abuse talking again." Oftentimes, clients who were hurt when younger did not have ways to fix, solve, or deal with the situation, so they become resigned to the fact that they are stuck and damaged or it must be their fault. "I am no good" is the mantra that repeats in their head.

It is fascinating to see how they think this way as a child, and then carry on those thoughts as an adult. They did not make the connection that it is the abuse that taught them that mantra, and it is not in fact true. As we know, abuse is never caused by the victim. It is all about the inflictor. The inflictor is not at all thinking of the victim, but the victim learns wrongly that it is about them and makes false conclusions about their worth. Correcting this idea and theme provides a new world-view in which the client is no longer subject to the abuse or its effects.

THEME: CARE TOO MUCH / PUT SELF LAST

Caring too much for others does not sound like it would be a problem. How can it be bad to help people? After all, is this not what therapists do? How can helping people be a theme that can cause difficulties with people? The problem surfaces when caring too much results in putting oneself last, and a person not setting healthy boundaries. These types of clients are more than willing to not only help others, but to help them at the expense of their own wellbeing. It is one thing to take a back seat and help someone else, but it is entirely different to stay in the back seat all the time. Clients struggling with this theme tend to talk about feeling empty, depressed, lost, and unimportant. If you listen, you will tend to hear frustration and anger coming from not feeling good or positive. Often, this is due to a person trying to help people when they are totally empty. I often explain this to clients using a story. We start with the premise that they are a kind person who enjoys helping people. People with this theme often say that they get enjoyment from helping, but they are no longer feeling enjoyment. The story goes like this:

> Imagine you only have enough money to fill up your car with enough gas to get you to work and back and each day. You only have the ability to fill up just enough to get through the day. So you are filling your daily allotment one day, and a friend shows up at the gas station and says, "Can you help me? My car is broken and I need to get to my job it is very important and if I am not there today I will not get paid."

> You know you only have enough gas for one trip. So you ask where she works and see that it is only a mile away from where you were going. You like to help people, so you say, "Fine." As you think in your head how you will have to walk from where she works, but if you go fast you will only be about 15 minutes late for work and you can make that up over lunch. You do that, and walking back to your car that night you are frustrated, tired and feel bad. Imagine how your reaction would be different if when you are at the gas station, you are filling up your entire tank and your friend asks for a ride. Notice how things are different. You not only offer to take her to work but will pick her up after work and bring her to her car, help her get groceries, and help anything else that she needs. While driving home after dropping her off at her car and helping her with rides, you feel good and were glad you were in a spot to help her. Why the difference in reactions? Your tank was full.

This is what we are talking about when clients keep putting themselves last. They wonder why are they not feeling better when they are helping people. The tricky part of the story is: How do you get in a spot to fill your tank up? You have to say no sometimes to the person asking for ride. If you are not able to do so, that is an issue. By setting a boundary and taking care of yourself, you will be able to feel better and retain your ability to help people in a manner that helps them and you.

OTHER THEMES

As therapists grow in their profession, they will continually identify new themes common in their clients. Some examples include control, fear of being alone, and the need for acknowledgement. Therapists will also come across very specific individually based themes that show up on a more personal level. An example of this would be specific triggers in PTSD cases.

New therapists often feel pressure to find themes, but it is clearly something for which you can't plan ahead. If you let people talk long enough, a theme will surface. It's important for new therapists to resist the urge to move too quickly in an attempt to fix the initial problem at the expense of taking enough time to hear the client share things that will help identify a theme. Once you hear and recognize a theme, you will be amazed how it will show up in almost every session. When clients talk about the incidents that have occurred, the theme becomes evident in a lot of their conversations. If you can begin to listen for themes, you will have a clear goal and purpose to your counseling, and it won't feel as though you are simply jumping from problem to problem.

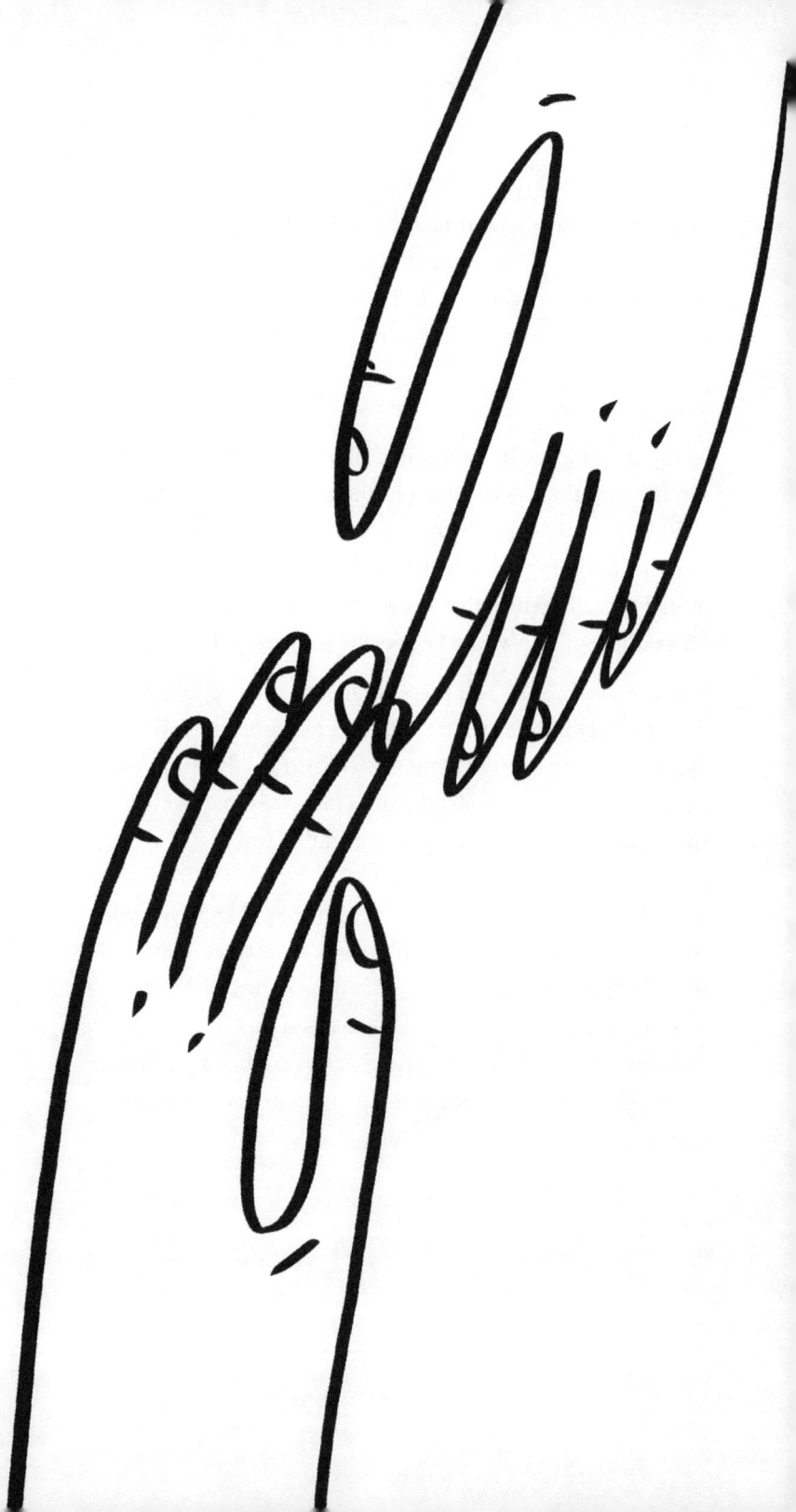

Marital Themes

MARITAL THEMES

There are a number of themes that you will begin to recognize when working with marriages. Working with marriages is a lot more difficult, as there are many sides and emotions coming out all at once. Slowing these emotions down to sort them out can be difficult, but it's imperative. When identifying marital themes it is important to differentiate them from the individuals themes that will also be present. (They are all operating at the same time.)

Being able to label something as a marital theme will help the couple begin to see what they need to work on and notice how their individual themes interact with their marital themes. I will frequently label marital themes as "we" problems. Helping them work on a "we" problem is often better than starting to work on two individual "me" problems. Pointing out this "we" problem in their marriage is beneficial as it allows each spouse to let down their guard and begin to work on something without feeling too defensive. Often there are "me" problems to work on within the marriage, but it is helpful to get them to agree that they both want to work on the marriage, or the "we."

Let's explore a few general themes that show up in marital counseling.

▶THEME:◀ NOT IN LOVE

As marriage counselors, we often here one spouse proclaim that they are not "in love" anymore. Allowing the spouse who feels this way to speak can be difficult, especially when the other spouse is sitting in the same room, upset and hurting. It is tempting to try to defuse the situation and move the conversation into a more positive direction, but it is particularly important to try to help the partner articulate what they mean by not being or feeling "in love."

Do you, as a therapist hearing this, know what they mean? Do they know what they mean? There can be a multitude of different reasons why someone gets to the point of being "not in love," but you want to spend some time trying to get them to articulate what that means to them. Often, the person saying that they are not in love anymore has difficulty explaining exactly what that means. They don't have difficulty telling you how they got there and all the problems they have had as a couple along the way. It is usually fairly easy for a frustrated spouse to share their anger and disappointment. It is much harder for a spouse to share feelings of loss for how they miss the relationship of which they used to be a part.

When you hear a theme of "not in love," it will tend to sound like a list of frustrations about or failures of the other spouse.

If you can have the hurting spouse share the hurt and not the anger, you begin to learn if there is any hope for saving the marriage. If the hurting spouse can talk about the loss of the dream or missing their spouse, you have some potential to work with them. If all you are hearing about is that the love is gone and they don't really care anymore, it becomes a little more dicey to try to save the marriage. If they say the love is gone, try to reframe the statement to ask if they are open to the possibility that they could be in love again. They most likely will be resistant and talk about all the things that need to change and how things were so bad that they are not sure they could ever love that person again.

Keep it on the theme of "not in love," not on that individual person and their flaws. Are they willing and do they want to be in love again—not necessarily with their current spouse but with anyone? If the answer is, "Yes," then you can begin to challenge them with the tasks of what it takes to be in love. Getting them to shift from their spouse as the problem to, "Are you willing to look at what you need to do to be in love?" is the theme with which you are trying to help. Start by going through a list of skills of what it takes to fall in love and ask if they have been doing those things.

If things are really dicey and it looks as though the marriage is most likely going to fail, it may force you to be more direct in your approach. If you don't have much time with a relationship you can afford to be bolder with your interventions. You may have to point out to the hurting spouse that they are half of the reason why they do not feel in love and they need to do things differently and learn new skills, so why not practice them with their current spouse regardless of if your marriage lasts? With this theme in marital therapy, you are simply trying to assess whether they are here to try and address things and work or whether they are looking for you to bless the failure of a dying marriage.

The same tactic is also taken with the spouse who has not "fallen out of love." Asking them how they got there can be enlightening. Are they taking all the blame in a desperate move to save the marriage? Are they putting all the blame on their spouse for not trying harder? Much like the "not in love" spouse, they typically have an easy time telling you their perspective of the marriage but have a much harder time telling you how serious and committed they are to trying to save it.

Pose similar questions around the theme such as, "Are you willing to do things differently even if your spouse does not want to?" and "What are you willing to do?" The theme of not being "in love" is typically about connection or not connecting. Are you "in love" with the handsome guy walking down the street? You may be attracted to him, but you are not "in love." Why not? I will heighten that scenario by asking a spouse in a more straightforward simple way, "Would you have sex with that guy walking down the street?" I usually get a horrified reply of "No. I don't even know him!" Well, that answer works for those who have fallen out of love. When you don't know someone, it is hard to be in love with that person.

Getting to know your spouse takes work. I often tell couples that I know it sounds scary when your spouse says that they don't love you anymore. I tell them that does not scare me. What will scare me is if your spouse says we are communicating, talking and sharing and I also don't think I love her. Knowing and loving go hand in hand. Addressing this theme involves assessing and seeing if the spouses are ready and willing to get to know each other again. Basically, are they willing to fall in love again? Or, taking a more realistic approach, I will ask, "Are you willing to get your heart broken again by your spouse?" This does not sound good, but that is the type of commitment you need to fight your way to a new and healthy marriage.

THEME: WE JUST DON'T COMMUNICATE

The next big theme you hear in marriage counseling is that we "just don't communicate." It is pretty standard rhetoric in all marriages and marriage therapy, and it is accurate. Communication and communication errors are a part of all marriages. The damage that poor communication causes can be devastating and kill a marriage. When a spouse says, "We don't communicate anymore," it is actually a false statement as they are still communicating messages, but they most likely are not the accurate ones. It may have deteriorated to the point of almost only body language, but it is still communication.

This theme sometimes is clearly stated using the actual words of, "We don't communicate," and other times it will come out in a variety of different ways that are not as clear. A spouse will say things like, "He never listens to me," "She does not care what I think," or "I know what she is going to say." All of these are just illustrations of the theme of communication struggles. A spouse usually listens, does care, and does not always know how their spouse will respond, but it is usually not done in the way they had hoped. How they said it and how it was heard often are two different things. The best way to address this theme is to slow them down so they can be more direct and authentic in what they are trying to communicate. An idea gets lost because what is being asked or what is needed is unclear. Couples will often hide their true feelings or the level of their true feelings in details that are not important. The couple ends up arguing or discussing the details and missing the point (feeling), or they end up ignoring the details and missing the point. Here's an example:

Wife: "You never listen to me when I tell you to do things around the house. Yesterday, I asked you to load the dishwasher and you didn't. All you did was sit and watch TV."

Husband: "That is not true. I did not watch TV all night. I drove the kids to practice, paid the bills, and I was going to load the dishwasher, but you were still in the kitchen."

Wife: "I never said you watched TV all night. I know you picked up the kids, but that was because I was doing the laundry. So you can't load the dishwasher while I am in the kitchen?"

Husband: "No. I can't, because you will just criticize and show me how to load it the right way."

Wife: "Well if you don't get things in there correctly, they don't get clean and then it is even harder for me to clean later, making more work for me."

That is a typical conversation in which there are way too many details and distractions. Can you spot the feeling? She did not share it very clearly and it was at the end of all talking. Look at the first sentence. Why is she asking him to do things around the house? Look at the last sentence. Why is she complaining about more work for her? She is clearly overwhelmed and needing some help, as she is struggling with all the work that she has to do. What is the feeling she is trying to communicate? It is most likely something along the lines of "I need some help because I feel that there is too much work for me right now."

If she casually says, "Can you load the dishwasher later?" the importance of how helpful this would be for her and why she needs it can easily get missed. If she shares her feelings by saying, "I am feeling overwhelmed and can't do everything. Can you help me?" it is less likely to get missed and will be heard by her husband. Helping couples communicate is all about getting the right, authentic, real feelings across to the spouse, and then making a response.

THEME: AFFAIRS

Unfortunately, another common theme you will come across in marital therapy is the issue of affairs. Numerous books have been written on all the intricacy and effects of affairs, as it inflicts a dramatic and devastating blow to a marriage. There are too many things to fully discuss when talking about affairs, but there is one basic theme of which you need to always be aware. When you have a couple in your office and you are working on things, both you and the clients need to know what you are talking about in the session—the affair or the marriage.

Those are two separate issues that obviously need to be talked about, but couples who are in crisis tend to try to do both at the same time. They will start talking about the affair and end up talking about their marriage, which unfortunately makes things very convoluted. If the person who had the affair thinks they are talking about the marriage, they will share their frustrations about the marriage and it will look like they are blaming a spouse for why they cheated. Or conversely, if the offended spouse thinks they are talking about the affair he will be quiet, not saying much. But if the other spouse thinks she is talking about the marriage, she will make the conclusion that he does not care about the marriage, as he is not saying anything.

If done correctly, both spouses will know what topic is being discussed. If it is the affair, the conversation will be one sided with the offended spouse expressing their hurt, anger, and devastation and the offending spouse accepting responsibility for what happened. If they are talking about the marriage it will be more of an equal amount from both parties talking about how or what they would like different in the marriage. As a therapist you need to be acutely aware of which one you are talking about to direct the conversation in the right manner. Often couples will switch back and forth frequently when they in the beginning stages of trying to deal with an affair.

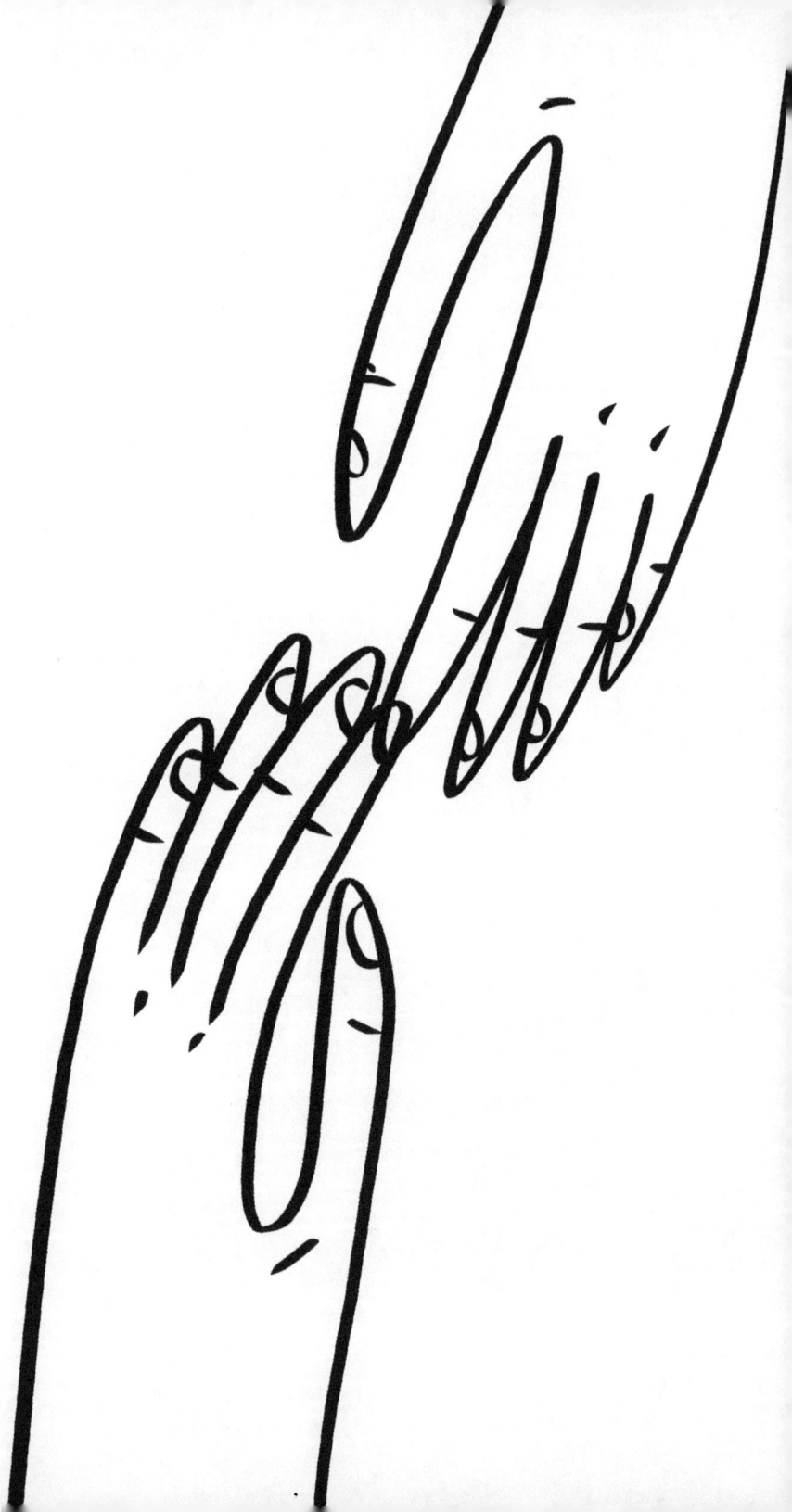

Kid Themes

THEMES COMMON WITH KIDS

Identifying themes is a more difficult task when working with children. Kids tend not to tell you how they feel, but they will show you how they feel. You have to gather a lot of collateral information from others to be able to identify the themes. I will talk more about how to work with kids more specifically in a later section.

THEME: SAFE AND SECURE

It's important that we as child therapists remain on the lookout for the common theme of a child not feeling safe and secure. Identifying such a theme can be challenging, as parents will be quick to point out all of a child's negative behaviors but not equate the behaviors with that child not feeling safe and secure. Children who struggle to feel safe often display a number of behaviors that include defiance and anger, and they can even exhibit some self-destructive behaviors. Attachment issues are most commonly associated with adoption, but they can surface in all families, especially if the environment is chaotic early on in the child's life. Early childhood trauma can also prevent a child from feeling safe and secure.

When beginning therapy with a child, it is tempting to start addressing negative behaviors without fully knowing their cause, but it's important that we take a more careful approach. Simply treating symptoms is never a good idea. Finding out what is going on or what happened can take a little digging. My experience has taught me that families often will overlook or not put enough importance onto feeling safe and secure for strong attachments to occur.

Frequently, when I am doing an intake and I am hearing about all the things that this child is doing, I will have this feeling that none of this makes sense. If I am having difficulty finding a cause for all these behaviors, I will ask some more probing questions, typically something as simple as, "Anything else I need to know about you that is unique or different?" Almost always, I will hear some type of story about how the child experienced some type of trauma or hurt. Parents will say that it happened a number of years ago and the child has adjusted well and moved on from that. For example:

> **Therapist:** "Anything else important, different or unique that I need to know about you?"

> **Parent:** "I don't know. . . . Oh, I just should let you know that she is not my biological daughter. She is technically my niece. Her mother was not taking care of her and doing drugs and she was at Grandma's a lot. She would frequently come to our house and play with my kids, and then over time

she just stayed with us. That was when she was four, so that was ten years ago and we just view her as part of the family."

Therapist: "Wow that is definitely a unique story. What do you want to add to that?" (Directing the question at the child.)

Kid: "Yeah, I don't think about it too much anymore."

The first lesson in life that this child learned was that she was not valuable and she does not matter. Even if the first lesson you learn is wrong, it can sometimes take a lifetime to learn differently. But for the therapist, knowing this fact sheds new light on the behaviors and how to address them.

If the parents are unaware of how this child struggles with not feeling safe and secure and the child is not overtly expressing these feelings, it can create a very wild situation. You must examine the times when the child is not feeling safe and talk about that instead of simply addressing the behaviors. If you want more information on attachment, please look up Karen Purvis at Texas Christian University and the Child Development Institute, who has some excellent information on the topic.

THEME: WORRY / ANXIETY

Kids carry lots of fears, some of them rational and some of them irrational. Children worry about storms, bugs, germs, and even sharks jumping out of the toilet! (Yes, that was an actual fear!) Many fears tend to be irrational, make no sense, or are not likely to occur. And typically, they will originate from something that is rational or based in reality such as getting abused, teased, or bullied. These reactions often tend to be out of proportion in relation to the actual risk.

Recognizing these fears is not too difficult, and this is one of the few times in which kids in therapy will tell you why they are here and what they need to work on. They often have been dealing with these issues for quite some time. Recognizing them is easy, dealing with them is not. Often, but not always, you will be able to recognize from where this excess worry or anxiety is learned or even taught. Frequently, one or possibly both of the child's parents will have a worrisome personality, if not an actual anxiety issue. Kids with anxiety, more often than not in my experience, have learned their worry from a parent. There can be a genetic component to this as well.

Some of these fears can result from a parent simply wanting to help their child prepare for every contingency or situation. They unintentionally end up alerting them to scenarios and possibilities of which they would not have otherwise thought. Parents, in trying to help, sometimes give their kids more things to worry about. A parent's concerned statement to a child about lightning can cause an irrational fear. Here is an example of conversation between a 10-year-old child and his parent that can lead to anxiety if the parent is overly anxious:

Child: "Can I go and play at Johnny's house."

Parent: "Sure. Just keep an eye out for thunder and lightning as it looks like it could storm."

Child: "Storm? Should I stay home?"

Parent: "No. Pay attention to the weather, because you want to be safe. You always want to be aware of the weather. You don't want to get caught in a thunderstorm, as you could get hit by lighting."

Child: "Hit by lightning?"

Parent: "Yeah. It will kill you. Lots of people get hit by lighting every year. You need to be careful and pay attention to when it starts to thunder, then get inside and be safe. Storms can be very dangerous and cause damage to houses and people."

Child: "Am I safe in the house during a storm?"

Parent: "Yes. But you should stay away from windows and electric outlets as sometimes when lightning hits a house the electrical wiring can start on fire."

Child: "Where is the safest place to be in a storm?"

Parent: "Usually in the basement."

Child: "I think that I will stay here instead of going to my friend's house.

Now, here are a few things to consider about this conversation. If a parent reviews this every time it could rain, it will add to the negative internal dialogue that is running through the child's head. If a version of this conversation happens repeatedly for a while, a bad pattern develops. A parent will think they are educating and helping a child, but they are actually reinforcing anxious thoughts. Fast forward to a year and now when the child is being brought in for anxiety and is asked about fears that he may. I might hear something like this:

Therapist: "Does he have any overreactions to certain things where you will see this anxious behaviors?"

Parent: "He refuses to go outside if there are a lot of clouds outside. He is fearful of storms. He is always asking about the forecast and if there are going to be any storms. If a storm actually happens, he is quite anxious and is telling everyone that they need to be in the basement and stay away from windows. He will get so anxious that he will refuse to go upstairs if it is raining outside. He always asks a lot about the forecast and the weather."

Therapist: "What do you tell him when it is storming?"

Parent: "Well I tell him that it is not a bad storm, and I will let him know if it is a bad storm and we need to go to the basement and take cover. I try to answer all of his questions so he can be know what is going on and can be aware of things."

Therapist: "What kinds of questions does he ask about the weather?"

Parents: "Well, he is pretty anxious, so he asks a lot of questions about what lighting can hit and what happens if our house gets hit. Those types of things."

Therapist: "What do you tell him?"

Parent: "Well, I used to tell him what would happened and that if the house started on fire we have a plan to get out. He knows the fire plan and how to get out of the house. I told him that we have insurance and that we would be okay and could rebuild our house. Recently, I have just been telling it is okay and not that bad of a storm."

The parent's intentions are good, and knowledge about how to handle situations is helpful. But are you able to hear and recognize the worry in the parent and how that could create his concern about people being safe and knowing how to handle situations? I have had parents say to me, "I need to be honest with my children. I don't want to lie to them. They need to know what the world is like." Yes, that may be true, but not every day, all the time. The parent's worry has now transferred to the child, and oftentimes the child does not have an adult frame of reference. What I mean in this case is that a child does not know how often a house or person gets hit by lightning. He has not been in hundreds of storms with no problems like his parent has. The child's worry turns to anxiety, and the fear prevents the child form being able to function. The parent is frustrated by his refusal to go outside when it is cloudy but does not realize the source of the worries. A better way to handle the situation would be as follows:

Child: "Can I go to Johnny's and play?"

Parent: "Yes, but listen for me if you are outside. I may yell for you to come home, as it might storm and I don't want you out in the storm."

Child: "Okay."

You have just sent the same message that you don't want him out in the storm. It is your job as a parent to watch the weather and call in your child—not his. You did, though, begin to teach him that you do not want him out in storms. If instead of saying, "Okay," he asks why he can't be out in a storm, you have two choices: Tell him that it is not safe to be out in storms or tell him if he wants to go to his friend's house he needs to follow the rules.

This conversation provides another of example of that when you are working with children, you are often working and treating the parents right alongside the children. The parents are the ones who are going to be doing things differently, not just the child. Helping both the parent and the child learn and identify what are kid worries and what are adult worries will be a reoccurring lesson with this type of theme. Often, kids worry about things that should be outside their concern—money, food, or housing. Those are not kid worries. Parents need to remind children that kids need to worry about their own much simpler issues, such as what to watch on TV or what games they want to play. Those are the things that should occupy their minds.

THEME: SELF-HARM / HURTING

It's a given that we're going to encounter kids who are hurting. In fact, most people in counseling are hurting in one way or another. What is different about this theme in children is that their internal hurt can lead to them outwardly hurting themselves. This outward expression of the hurt that they are feeling can be the reason they are brought to counseling. Kids with this theme tend to have been "caught" or discovered that they are hurting themselves.

There are lot of different ways in which kids hurt themselves, and some are more destructive, scary and in-your-face while others are quiet hidden and small. Some examples include cutting or hurting themselves, not eating, over exercising, or other punishing habits. Begin to address this theme by helping kids learn to identify what triggers their need to punish themselves or why they feel as though they deserve to be punished. Help the child first figure out the thoughts associated with the behavior, then focus on behavior modifications needed to stop the behavior. Spend as much time as you can on the thoughts and feelings to achieve better success in changing the behaviors.

THEME: I DON'T MATTER

One final child therapy theme that I would like to address is one that is hard to identify and is not always the initial reason for why a child would go to therapy—the theme of a child who feels as though they don't matter or are not loved. This differs from simply not feeling safe and secure. It does not necessarily involve past trauma or hurt, but it could be that they feel as if they are forgotten or have no support.

A child dealing with this issue might have been brought in for some type of negative behaviors, but the root of those negative behaviors could be negative-attention seeking. The child feels that any type of attention is better than nothing. When they display the behaviors, they at least feel as though they matter. This theme is often secondary, as the parents did not bring in the child to help them feel more important or to matter, but it is often underlying to the presenting behaviors. When this theme is present, it is often hard to get the parents to change their behaviors as they are blinded by the surface negative behaviors in the child. They see the symptoms, not the cause. They tend to resist this idea, as to them it feels as though they child is getting rewarded with more time when they are acting poorly. It takes some practice and clear explaining to help the child and the family move to a more loving and healthy feeling of support.

Kids themes are not much different than adult ones. Just remember that with kids, it takes more time to build trust, more time to identify underlying themes and more time to bring about change.

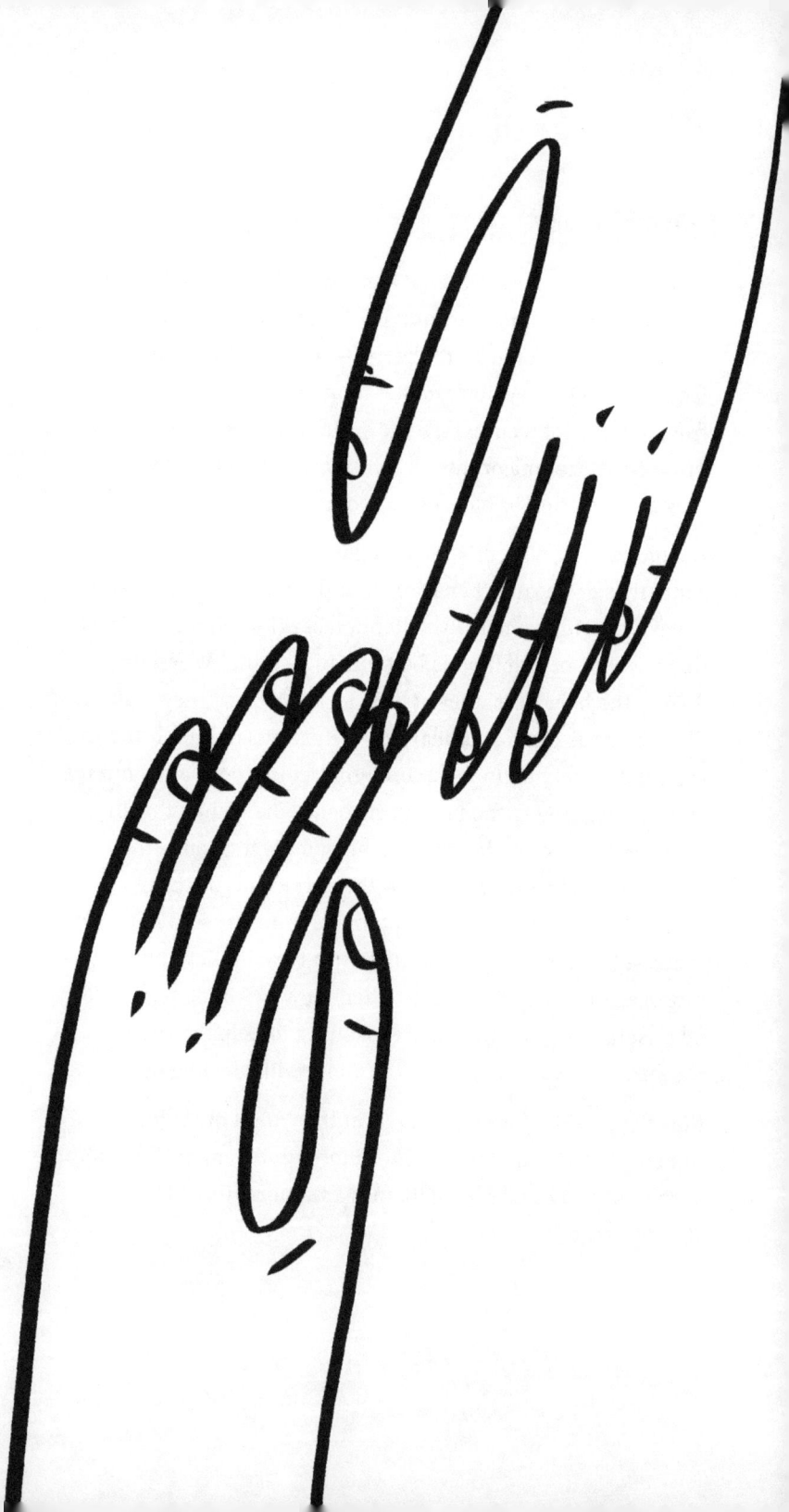

SECTION I: PART XI

Therapist Themes

THERAPIST THEMES

We have talked about common themes in individuals, marriage, children, but now we have to address one more area within the realm of themes. What are yours? What are some typical themes that therapists have or have to deal with?

What type of therapist are you? I'm not asking if you're a cognitive-behavioral or object-relations or narrative therapist—those are theoretical orientations. I want you to think about what type of therapist you are from a personality perspective.

Are you an anxious therapist, worrying a lot about your clients and what they are doing? Are you worried about how your clients are viewing you? Are you a pleasing therapist, wanting to make sure your client always feels good when leaving your session? Do you take too much ownership of their problems? Is it difficult to set strong boundaries with them? Do you always let them dictate when the session ends? Are you confrontational with them, challenging them to do better or be different.

Are you organized, always knowing what you are going to be addressing in session? Do you need to have a plan and a goal before each session? Are you disorganized and simply fly by the seat of your pants and see where the session goes?

These are all things that you need to know about yourself as a therapist. I tried to give extremes on both sides of each possibility in an effort to help you see that you can't say, "No," to all of them! We as therapists have our own issues! If you are thinking that I am not too organized but I don't fly by the seat of my pants, you may be missing the point. (Maybe you are defensive!) The point is not to be perfect or even like Goldilocks ("Just right"). The point is for you be aware of which way you are leaning, so you know that you need to work on leaning the other way.

Too often, we are like our clients and we don't want to take a long hard look at who we really are and how we really operate. Often when we are asked these questions and forced to pick and acknowledge our shortcomings, we get uncomfortable and simply want to give a general statement and move on. Would you let your client do that about their themes and issues? Once you know what type of therapist you are, you can the next questions of, "What types of clients do you work best with? Which clients fit well with your theme of who you are as a therapist? Which ones don't? How far are you willing to change who you are to work with a particular client?" You can adjust to try and meet clients in a certain spot, but if you move too far you may lose your authenticity or confidence in what you are doing. And it will not go well.

Here's an example. I am not a highly structured therapist who has a clear plan of what we are going to be talking about each session. I do not give out a lot of workbook-type homework. I tend to focus more on the cognitive thoughts and feelings of clients, why they have those thoughts and feelings, and how they can change them. I am definitely an "in the moment" type of therapist. In fact, astute readers will be able to see that the majority of this book simply offers ways to get clients in those moments so we can get to work. So if this is who I am as a therapist, I tend to not to work very well with highly organized and structured type-A clients. I drive them crazy. I may alter my approach knowing that I may have to give really specific and detailed homework, but I am not going to find and make up a bunch of handouts for a client even if that is what he or she may want. When a client asks me for workbooks or other outside material to use during our treatment, I will probably challenge them to do that work and report back to me what they have learned or found. Some clients will embrace that; some find that annoying. If I get a sense that a client is highly organized, I will address that early on in our sessions or even in the first session to prevent that from becoming an issue. I will tell them this is how I operate and how I do therapy. I will point out things such as, "If you are looking for a therapist who has a 12-step plan and outline on how to handle this issue, I am probably not the therapist for you. I operate in the realm of feelings and making you feel uncomfortable so that we can examine those feelings in an effort to find new ways to change."

If a client is seeking that type of therapist or is willing to try, we will be okay. If not, I am okay referring that client to a therapist who is more organized and structured. You will help your client more quickly and save some frustration for both if you acknowledge this extreme difference.

We can also get in touch with who we are as therapists by examining our approach to different therapy techniques. Some will fit your approach well, some will make you feel too uncomfortable, and some may not match well with who you are as a therapist. There has been a lot of research done on Eye Movement Desensitization and Reprocessing (EMDR), which is used to help people with trauma. The process involves putting clients through bilateral sensory input (such as having their eyes look at moving lights) while having them process traumatic events. It has been proven to be beneficial and healing with a number of issues, and I have had clients ask if I could do that with them. Why would I not learn how to do something that has been proven to help people if I am in the business of helping people and my clients are asking for it? Because it does not fit me, my style, or my theme of how I conduct therapy. There is nothing wrong with EMDR and I don't have any objections to it, and I have even recommended that some clients try it. EMDR simply does not fit my personality or how I approach or work best in therapy sessions. I could probably learn how to do it, but I am not sure that I would comfortable addressing traumatic situations with this approach. It does not fit my theme of who I am as a therapist, and I don't want to be unauthentic while trying to teach my clients to be authentic.

Another way to look at your therapist themes is to ask your clients what they see and notice. How would your clients describe you? How they perceive you can not only be enlightening but also helpful. Do they see you as caring, strong, that you've got it all together, or that you are struggling? Do they feel they're your equal or are you the expert?

Answers to such questions can be enlightening, as they can help you learn to see how you are perceived. Is it how you intend? It's good to know if a client is getting an entirely different message than the one you thought you are sending. And, if it is entirely different from what you have heard from other clients, what is going on there? Is this example of your client misreading you in a manner similar to times when they misread others? Do they overreact on miscommunications or always have a negative perception of themselves or others? Could that be part of what led them to counseling? You now have a great example with which to work and might have uncovered a new issue for therapy. Discussing your clients' perceptions of you can be beneficial and offer a great way to gather perspective.

It is also helpful to ask your client what they learned from their last therapist. Can they articulate that? What things did they like in therapy and what things didn't they not like? Are you able to adjust to what your client found beneficial, or is it too far out of your comfort zone? Knowing your themes as a therapist will help both you and your client get more out of sessions.

WHAT DOES A GOOD SESSION LOOK LIKE?

I often hear therapists I am supervising say things such as, "My last session with this client was really good," or, "That session was terrible." I often have those same feelings. With some sessions, I feel as though they went really well, while with others I might feel they fell short. Sometimes I think I am an awesome therapist and other times I think maybe I should just try a new career!

What causes those feelings in therapists? It is beneficial and necessary to identify what types of sessions feel good to you and which ones don't. When you finish a session and say, "That was a good session," what happened that made you feel good? In deciding what makes a good session and what makes a bad session, it is helpful to look at them in two different ways: What do you do in a session, and what does your client do in a session?

Did you have a good session based on things that you did? Did you make a good point or make a connection between your client's behaviors and thoughts? Were you able to link that in a manner that the client was able to see how they were having a dysfunctional thought? Did you provide some particularly helpful education on an issue, prompting the client to learn something new and increase understanding? Did you provide reflective listening and allow your client to vent and be heard? Did you provide some confrontation or challenge a client to elicit some new growth? Did you help in decision-making and give your client some new pros and cons to think about? Did you celebrate a success and provide support?

All of these accomplishments can be part of a good session, and it is helpful to recognize what makes us feel good during a session. One therapist may love providing education and understanding to clients while another may like to challenge clients to think differently. Another therapist might simply enjoy sitting quietly and listening to others. Knowing where you fit in with these reactions helps you be aware of what you are doing or striving for, or perhaps what techniques you need to use more often. If you enjoy providing education, you will most likely do that more than you realize. If you like to challenge, you will probably challenge more than you are aware. Does that mean that is wrong? Nope, it's just awareness. Remember, what we are talking about are good sessions. We sometimes may do things that do not make us feel good, but they may be, and probably will be, part of a good session.

On the client side, are there things your clients do or say to make a good session? When you walk out of a session and it feels as though it went well, was it based on what *they* told you? Did you hear compliments from them thanking you for what you have done for them? Did you say something that made sense to them and they were appreciative? Did you see learning in their face while you were talking that validated what you were thinking they needed to hear? Did you see relief in their face as the session progressed? It is helpful to think about the things your client does to make you feel as though you teamed up for a good session. Are you trying to create more of those experiences in your therapy? It is helpful to remember that these things may make *you* feel as though *you* just had a good session. But a good session to you and good session for your client can be two totally different things.

Remember who you are and recognize the things that motivate and please you. You obviously will not always have good sessions. You shouldn't always have good sessions. We are human, and we will have human reactions to how things go. But it is important for us to remember as therapists that therapy is never about us. Sure, we are allowed to have good sessions and we are allowed to feel good about what we do. If therapists never feel good about themselves in sessions, they are going to have long, rough, careers. But a session must always be, first and foremost, about the client. Keep the focus on them.

1. You are treating a 32-year-old married woman who came to you seeking help with self-esteem, confidence, and codependency issues. As she gets healthier, she is having more struggles with her husband who is not used to being with someone who is now speaking up and sharing opinions. The healthier she gets, the more dysfunction shows up in her marriage. Are you helping to break up a marriage?

2. You are treating a 16-year-old boy who is struggling with visitations he is having with his father. He shares how he has come to the conclusion that he does not want to have to keep going to his house for visitations since the visits are so pointless. Are you helping him articulate his feelings to his father and verbalize to his dad how he feels (sounds nice, huh?) or are you helping end a relationship between a father and son? (Not so nice!)

There are just a few examples of the thousands of types of scenarios that will occur. Do you find yourself wanting to know more about the husband in the above example, such as, "What type of person is he? Is he an alcoholic? Abusive? Is he kind, and is she now demanding that it be her way or she is leaving?" How about with example with the boy. "Is the dad someone who is never around on the weekends? Is he supposed to have his son yet frequently leaves him home alone, and the boy just wants to stay at his mom's house and not get emotionally hurt? Or, is mom trying to alienate a good father who is trying desperately to connect with his son because she is still bitter and willing to make her children suffer for their divorce?"

Now does having extra information help? Why? Does that information help you in how you help you client? Does the client still have the same choices regardless of whether the choice is good or bad? Can you still help the woman work through a divorce even if you believe the marriage has potential? Can you advocate for the boy even if his father is a "standup guy," so to speak? This is where it is important to remember a lesson we talked about earlier: What are you being hired to do?

As a therapist, you do not have to do every job your client wants you to do, but you need to be clear as to why you are not taking certain jobs. It should never be simply because you do not like what the client is choosing. No one ever said this was easy.

Here are some suggestions I have used to help me get through some of these dilemmas. I have found that if you do these things, they tend to help both you and the client see things more clearly. First, paint the picture. Clarify what they are asking you to do.

Good therapists are not always liked. My mother would occasionally tell me how she ran into someone who had seen me as a therapist. Sometimes they would know I was her son, sometimes not. She would always tell me, "Your clients seem to really like you. I can tell you are a good therapist." I would warn her and say, "Well, I hope now and then you will come across someone who does not like me, because that means I am being real and telling people things that they don't always want to hear." Sometimes a good session will not feel like a good session! Helping clients grow can cause growing pains, and sometimes they are not ready to grow. And sometimes, clients want to grow in the wrong way.

Lastly, when examining yourself as a therapist, ask yourself this question: Are you able to help a client choose a path that is not beneficial to them?

Therapy is about helping people. Can you help them make a dysfunctional or unhealthy choice? Client self-direction is important, ethical and hard. You need to be ready to help clients with their answers, not yours. We do not get to dictate how our clients should act, what they choose, or how they grow. They come in with a problem, and we offer ways to help them. They may not always choose our way to solve the problem. When faced with a situation or dilemma of a client making a bad choice to solve their dilemma, you cannot impose your will. Here are some interesting and sometimes difficult circumstances that you will face as a therapist:

> **Therapist:** "Are you asking me to help you eliminate all contact from your father?"
>
> **Boy:** "Well, maybe not all. I want to be able to call him if I want ,but I don't want to feel like I have to and I don't want to talk to him right now."
>
> **Therapist:** "What would be a situation in which you would want to call him?"
>
> **Boy:** "I don't know. Maybe if he wanted to actually do something with me."
>
> **Therapist:** "What would you like to do with him?"
>
> **Boy:** "I don't know."

I am ending the conversation here, as it does not matter what he wants to do. The conversation has just shifted from never wanting to visit his dad to needing to have a good reason to contact him. This is a much healthier conclusion, one that empowers him but also gives him room to operate in future situations. I can help him with that job. We will have to clarify how to talk to Dad, how to handle disappointment, how to make sure Dad understands him, what to do if Dad continues to emotionally disappoint, how to handle talking to Mom about maybe wanting to have some type of contact. These are all things I like and can do as a therapist. Paint the picture so you have a clear understanding of what kind of help for which your client is really asking. Make the statements bold so you can clarify their expectations. Finally, allow room to explore their answers.

Another tip for clarifying your clients' asks involves keeping things simple. When the woman in the above example states that she is frustrated with the new frequent arguments she is having with her husband, you can go beyond simply pointing out that this may be a result of her addressing and setting boundaries. Asking her, "Do you think your marriage will survive in its current condition?" is a simple yet powerful question that you can now explore. Is she okay if her marriage ends? Does she want things to be better? Is it time for a new task for us in counseling, meaning that we had been working on setting boundaries but maybe now we need to shift to working on communication skills with her husband? Remember that these are all her choices, but stating things simply helps clarify a situation while allowing a client to choose his or her course of action.

Finally, you may have to help a client with a dysfunctional conclusion. If you have a highly anxious OCD client who is struggling to get control of things but states that he does not want to take medicine for it, you can agree. You will also want to say, "Okay. We will try to address this without meds, but if we find that after a few sessions we are not making any progress, can we revisit the medication issue and possibly try that?" You can help them try, even though you are well aware of the research and success rate of treating an OCD disorder without medication.

All of these are themes that warrant your attention. The themes are always there. They influence how you practice. Recognize, address, and manage them, rather than ignore them and pretend they don't exist.

Section II:
GETTING DOWN TO BUSINESS

TREATMENT: HELPING THEM CHANGE

Once you have made a solid connection with your client and helped them identify themes in their life, it is time to get down to work on helping them do things differently. Recognizing struggles or problems is one thing; implementing change is something different.

Doing things differently is a lot like learning to break a bad habit and replace it with a healthy one. It takes a lot of repetition to get to a point in which you are doing something without even thinking about it. There is a lot of research on how to change and fix bad habits. The general rule, which seems to make sense to me, is to focus on replacing the old way instead of simply trying to stop the old way. It's much easier to focus on what you are trying to do instead of focusing on what you are not trying to do is. This is similar to the old phrase, "Don't think about a big pink elephant." What are you thinking about now? A pink elephant! Too often, clients act in a similar manner as they have recognized their theme or dysfunctional thinking and they want to simply stop doing it. That is pretty hard to do if they don't in some way to do it differently. In this next section, we will look at helping clients learn to do this process on their own without always needing a therapist to point out when the dysfunction is happening and what to do with it. We will be looking at a couple different steps.

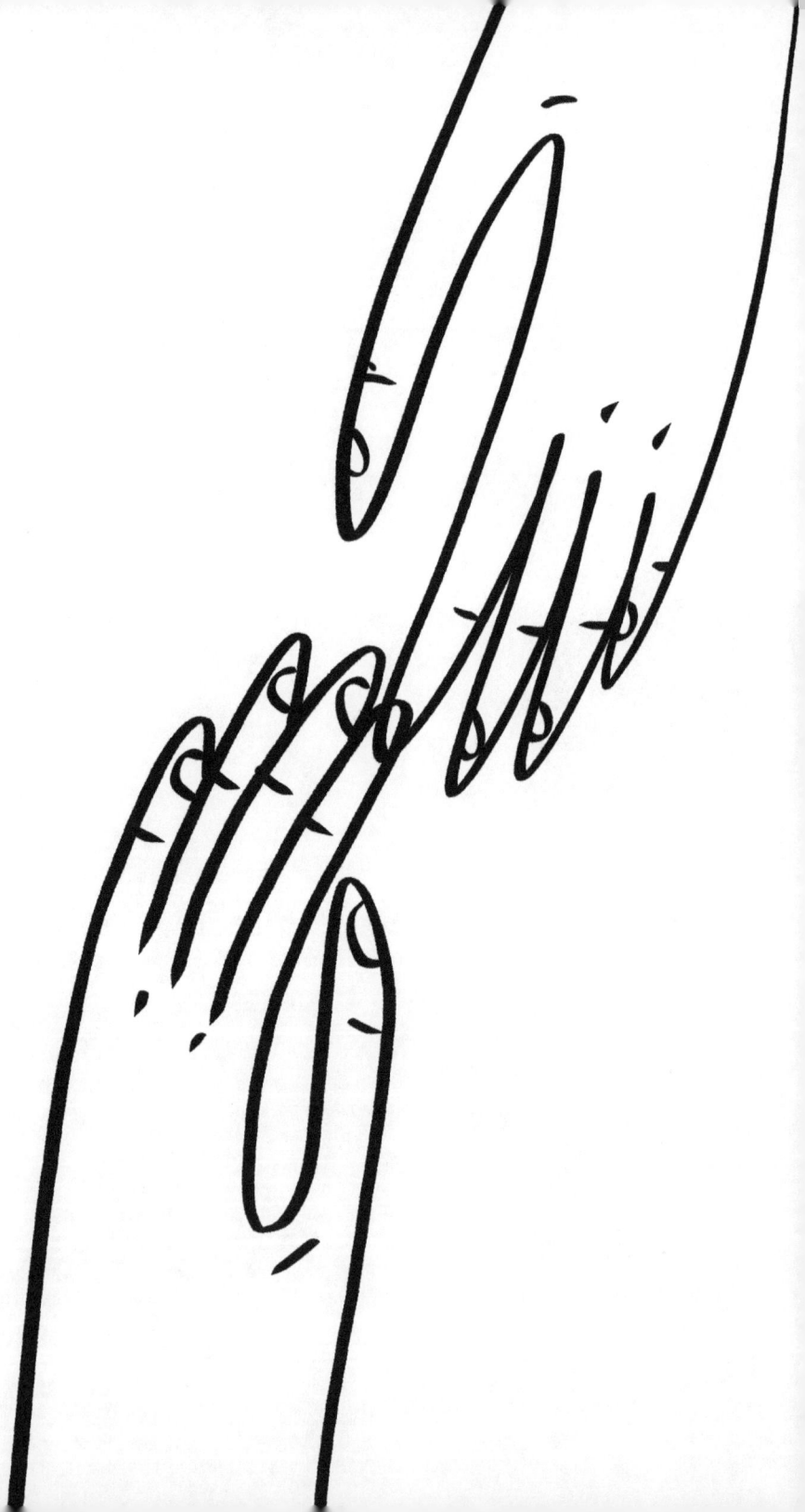

SECTION II: PART I

Awareness

AWARENESS

The first step in this process is to teach awareness to identify the issue. Clients need to be able to recognize on their own when the dysfunctional theme, idea, or coping skill shows up. This is a theme that you and your client have identified as an issue needing attention. You are trying to help them catch themselves before they start doing the same old thing. We have, up to this point, simply pointed out the theme, but it is important for the client to be able to find this theme on their own so that can begin to address it in real time. Teaching them to slow down to pay attention to their feelings is vital for them to identify and correct things. As clients get better at this, they will be able to tell you that they recognized the theme in the situation while it was happening. When they are able to do this, it allows the opportunity for change to happen.

Growing this awareness from the counselor's office to out in the real world often involves teaching your client to slow down.

Frequently, they are responding and reacting without much thought, as they have done this for years. Teaching them to slow down, be aware of what is happening, and ask themselves how they are feeling can do wonders. I will often have clients practice by asking themselves a couple times a day to simply check in and see how they are feeling. I ask them to practice taking some time to take an inventory of how they are feeling at a particular moment. They are not allowed to use feeling-neutral words such as "good," "fine," or "okay." Once they are better able to track their feelings, they are better able to identify when the change in feelings in occurring, which is a sign that the theme or dysfunctional response is happening.

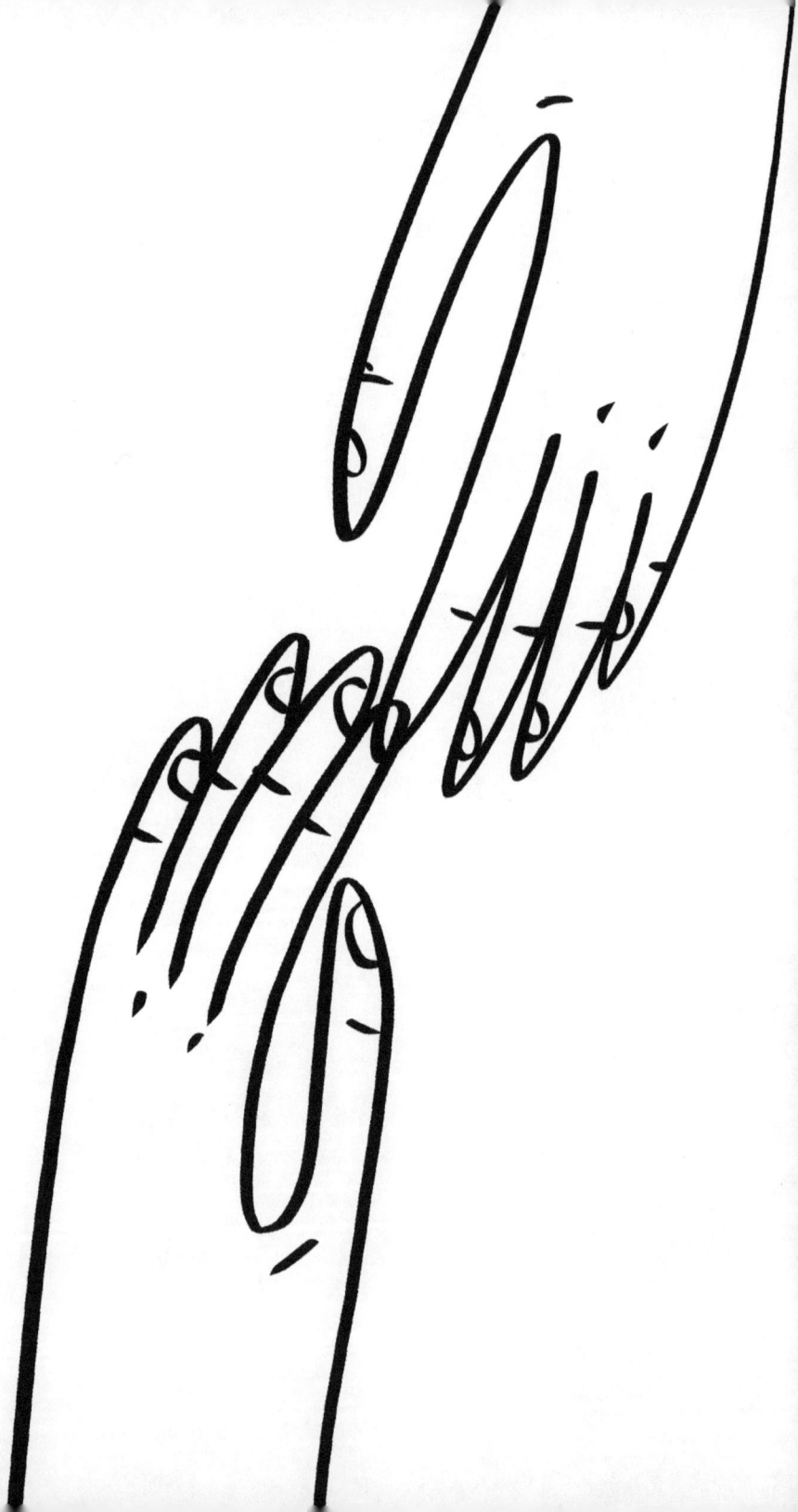

Implement

IMPLEMENT

The next step is to implement. After clients have identified that the same old pattern is occurring, they can actually implement some change on their own. Finally, they can do it differently. Clients need to have some choices or options about what they can do differently. This is where their homework comes in. Clients need to be able to know how to approach things differently, and they only know how to approach things differently through the homework you have assigned for practice. Keep things simple. There does not need to be a five- or ten-step process on implementing changed behaviors. They don't even have to know what to implement. Often, I will tell clients, "Just do something differently. What you have been doing is not working. Just change the pattern, and you will start new reactions and patterns that tend to be much more healthy." These are the steps of identify and implement. Be aware of what is going on, and then do things differently. Sure, it's simple, but remember the key to what we will be addressing is repetition and practice. We need to look at this a little deeper.

Now that your clients can recognize the feelings and identify when the "old' way of thinking starts, they need to make the change. These homework assignments not only help them reframe their perspective so they "see" the situation differently, but they also can take a different action than they have previously selected. Your client will initially struggle with identifying different ways of seeing or doing things. Give them clear homework to practice something new and differently.

Here is an example of how that would look in an individual session with a client who has identified a theme that she always put others before herself, which has caused her to stuff a lot of her feelings and leave her down and depressed. She is far enough along in the process that she has not only identified this, but she also believes it is true and contributes to her current level of depression.

Therapist: "So, did you have any times this week when you were experiencing some difficult feelings?"

Client: "Well, last night when I was getting ready for bed, my husband commented on how messy the bedroom was and that he would clean it up tomorrow. It made me mad, because he has been saying that same thing for the last three nights. I would just as soon hear him say nothing and just do it. Telling me that he is going to do it and then never do it is just frustrating, but I guess I should be grateful that at least he knows that it is something that bothers me and I would like it picked up."

Therapist: "Sounds as though you were a little annoyed at his comments. What did you do?"

Client: "Nothing. I wouldn't know what to tell him. I'm afraid that it would come out wrong and start a big fight at bedtime, and I don't want to do that. He always tells me that I get way too emotional over things. I am not sure how I would tell him."

Notice that the client has progressed in therapy and she was able to identify a situation or a time when she was upset, knows why she was upset, and is aware of how that fits into her thinking. She has this part down, but she does not know what to do next. She can recognize the issue, but she is not far enough along in the process to be able to implement something different.

Therapist: "Why don't you just tell him what you just told me? You explained it pretty well to me."

Client: "What? Just tell him that telling me he is going to do it and not do it is frustrating and just do it without telling me?"

Therapist: "Yep"

Client: "But what if he gets angry and tells me that I am being too picky and controlling."

This resistance is normal, and it provides a clue that you identified the correct thing, as her doing something differently is causing her to get nervous and scared. Your client is already nervous about sharing her feelings and the potential reactions she might get. If you were to give the assignment of, "Well, the next time you notice this feeling, just tell yourself it is not a big deal and try to move on with your night," your client would not resist and most likely would say, "Okay." She knows how to do this. This would be you simply asking her to do more of the same.

It is easy to do the same old stuff, and harder and riskier to do something differently. It is at this point that you will have to help your client remember the lessons you have covered. Keep it simple and direct—not a lot of facts—and keep the feelings basic and bold: "It is frustrating for me when you talk about picking up your clothes, but don't." If she adds much more, her spouse will miss that feeling and an argument will ensue.

She also needs to be reminded that her job is only to make that statement of feeling. Her job is not to be responsible for how her husband responds. Whether he says, "I am sorry for frustrating you. That is not what I am trying to do," or, "I can say and do whatever I want because this is my house, too, and there is nothing you can do about it," she is successful either way. She did something differently by sharing her feelings directly and calmly instead of stuffing and exploding. Success is dictated by what she does, not by the response she receives. Continuing on with the conversation:

> **Therapist:** "Remember, you are not responsible for his actions, just your part of saying things differently."

> **Client:** "Okay. The next time that happens, I will try to tell him."

Don't let the client off the hook right here. We are trying to do things differently. They need to learn to seek out situations to practice instead of hoping they remember next time.

Therapist: "Why don't you tell him about your feelings tonight when you get home? Don't wait 'til next time. Go seek him out.

You can be prepared, and it can happen on your terms when you are ready as opposed to you hoping to remember how to do this the next time it comes up."

This gives the client a little extra feeling of control and safety as they are just beginning to do things differently. Teaching them to seek out opportunities as opposed to waiting for them moves the process along at a greater pace.

Tell your clients to go easy on themselves, as often they will be halfway down the road of handling something the old way before they identify what is happening and realize that they are handling the situation in the same old way. You will need to remind the client that they may have to stop or even work their way backwards out of the old way of handling something in the beginning. Also, remember that clients may be doing well for a while, and then a bigger incident or crisis will occur and they will regress to their old ways of handling a situation. Help them rebound, and encourage them to practice, practice, practice.

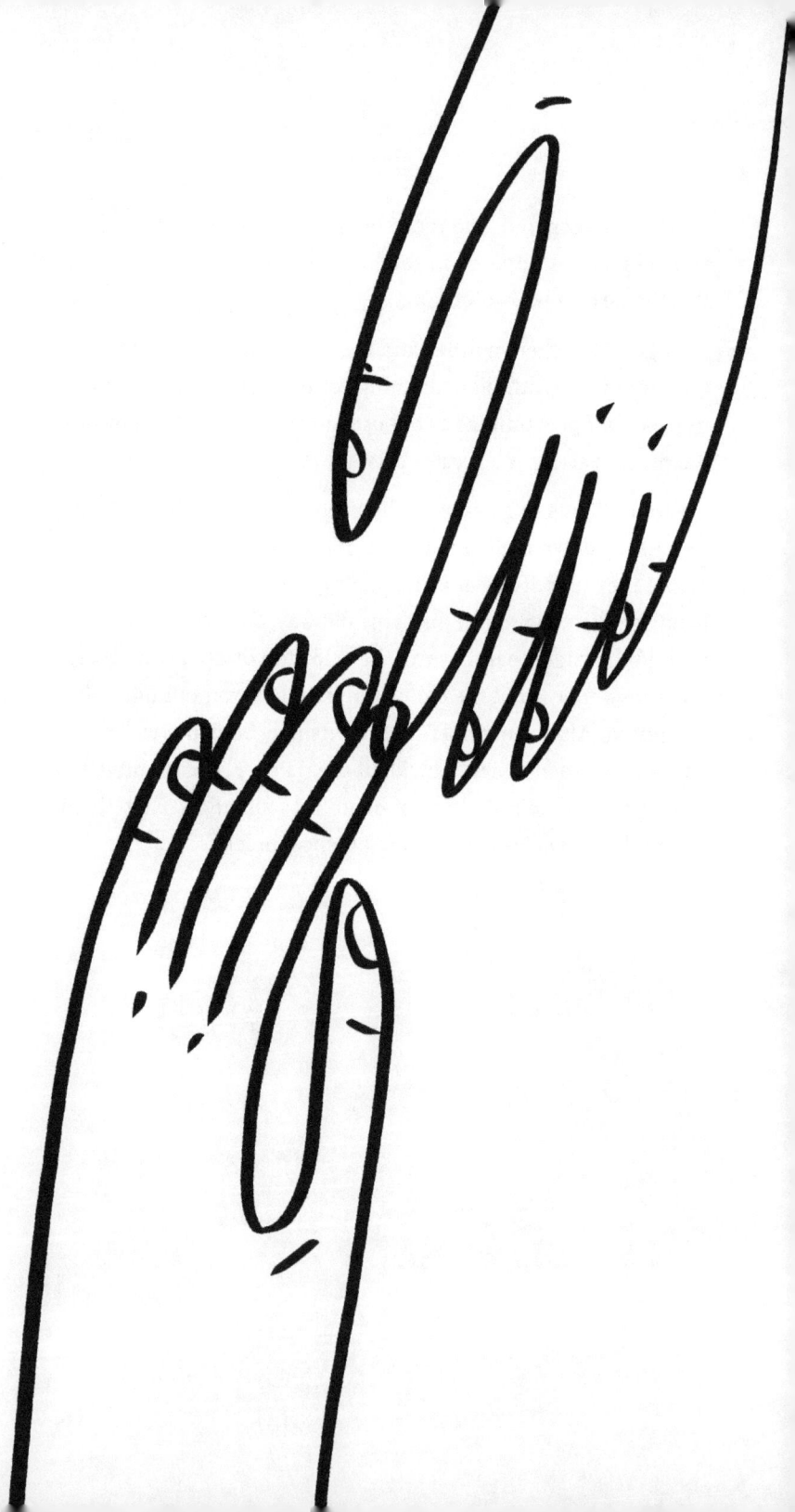

Homework and/ or teach them new responses

ENGAGING THEM IN NEW RESPONSES: HOMEWORK

Now that you have your client seeing and identifying that they need to do things differently, and they are willing to do things differently, you have to help them get there. This is where a good therapist earns his money! The homework needs to fit the situation.

"What is your plan?" I say this frequently in therapy, as clients will begin to accurately state what they are thinking and enumerate the problem, and then they stop talking. They get really quiet. They don't know WHAT to do differently.

Here is an example from a recent session. I had a client who was struggling with an eating disorder. We worked hard on trying to help her identify that she was avoiding her feelings and coping in a negative way by spending more time focused on her binging and purging than on the real problem. When I asked her what she was feeling when she needed to puke last night, she initially said she didn't not know. As we worked and talked about things, she first said that she was worried about financial things. Then, through therapy, we talked about needing to be more specific, as general is not always helpful, She then stated accurately, "Last night, I had to talk to my family because of our financial struggles. We are not able to go on a family vacation as we had planned, and that was difficult and hard for me to tell them as I felt like a failure."

"Perfect," I thought in my head. She identified the feeling, used words that fit her theme of a feeling like a failure, and it was a specific incident. She had developed and applied a sense of insight into what was occurring. I then asked her about her plan to do things differently instead of purging when she feels like a failure. "I have no idea," she said. This is what I mean when I say clients get quiet. We went on to talk about the different things she can do or ways to handle that feeling.

Making the connection that purging does not help ease her feeling that she is a failure is helpful, but we need to help her with what does help the feeling. We talked about simply enduring the feeling and doing nothing, as it is temporary and inaccurate. We talked about making plans to rectify the situation to save for a family vacation. We talked about being able to do something smaller, etc. These are a variety of things with which you and your client can brainstorm to develop alternative healthy coping skills. Here is where you can use the wealth of information that is already out there: books, articles, workshops, other therapists' ideas, your techniques, systems, or theories. This is where all of those different theories of change come into play. You can finally start to use whatever theory you have been trained in.

TAKE SOME TIME

Take special note about how far we are in the process with our client. You are significantly far into this book (almost done!), and we are just now talking about doing things differently. This is what most people think is the regular part of therapy. . . change. This is just another reminder of the importance of connection and identifying the problem. If you go to fast, you start working on change and the client is not invested into the process. They may feel temporary relief, but not lasting change. You then actually become just another negative coping skill they have learned to use. The client learns, "When I am overwhelmed, I go talk to a therapist and I feel better." They don't know why or how it works, but they feel better, then they drop out only to repeat the pattern the next time they are overwhelmed. Therapy works for a while, but they do not know why they are doing what they are doing, and it unfortunately becomes just like the woman who was purging. She doesn't know why she is doing what she is doing.

Therapy is similar. When you ask a client after a few sessions why they are coming in and what specifically they are working on with you, you may hear things like, "You are trying to help me feel better." If that's the response, you have failed. You want to hear things such as, "You are helping me learn how to handle my feelings of failure in a better way." Too often, hurting clients are used to making dysfunctional choices or using poor coping skills, and you can fall right into the trap. Therapy can become a poor coping skill as well. We have all made the mistake of letting a client get into the routine of coming in and telling you all the bad things that happened during a particular week, then giving them a few supportive comments before sending them on their way . . . only to repeat the process in two weeks. This is what I mean by adding to the negative-coping-skill process.

Remember, most of therapy is helping people identify the dysfunctional thoughts and letting them see that more often than not, there are not as many problems as they think—just negative ways of handling normal life events. The feelings they are experiencing probably should be there. They may not "feel" good, but they are healthy and the negative feelings are most likely temporary. A client will feel lonely at times. That is not a problem or even something that needs to fixed immediately. But if a client takes that feeling of loneliness, thinking there is something wrong, it quickly goes from, "I am lonely," to, "I am a loser." And when this happens, the client feels like a failure and may start to do things to try and fix their issues in ways that are not always healthy. Counseling is about helping people understand that they are okay—they are lonely and okay, they are sad and okay, etc. Therapy is about helping them address and endure the lonely, not fix the feeling that they are a failure. That is the theme you are trying to correct, and I know of no better or more efficient way to help clients know that they are okay than highlighting to them that God sees them as okay!

HOW DID THEY GET LOST?

How do your clients get here? How did they learn these negative coping skills? Why don't they have positive ones?

Unfortunately, they don't know any better, and they don't know any different responses. They are not always sure of the correct way to respond to the situation, as they have not seen many correct ways. They make mistakes because they have never been taught or shown correct and healthy ways. When learning about their themes, clients will discover how they have accepted or learned something that is not accurate. They will often feel ashamed and inferior as they grasp the concept and it becomes glaring obvious as to why they have been struggling. They will often say, "It is so simple. Why did I not recognize that? I should have seen that. I never thought of that, but when you point it out it seems so easy."

It is important that you help them understand that the reason they don't know is because they don't know! Replace their shame with optimism. Point out to them how they are great learners and respond to learning. You can often point out to them they have actually learned a lot on their own. People learn through trial and error or having a teacher *show* them so they can skip some of the errors.

How did you learn how to drive? First, you likely watched your parents drive thousands of times before you were allowed to try, giving you some 16 years of observation. Then you were given lessons by your parents or through driver's education classes. You are taught. Sure, teens still needs to practice, as the parent hopes that the learning and evolving of this skill does not involve too many dents or accidents.

Now, think about driving as an adult. Try to recall all the skills and steps that the task requires. Are you even aware of them? Just look at the steps of backing a car out of the driveway:

1. Stick key in ignition.

2. Turn the key.

3. Let key go once car is started.

4. Look in mirror to make sure nothing is behind you.

5. Place foot on brake.

6. Take car out of park and put in reverse.

7. Take foot off break and put on the accelerator.

8. Turn and look over shoulder.

9. Check side so you don't hit mirror going out of garage (that step gets missed sometimes ☺).

10. Proceed.

Did you think about each step, or did you just do them? That is the result of years and years of practice after being taught the steps. You now do them without even thinking. At this point (for most of us) backing out of the garage is easy. You would feel shame if you could not do it by now. The same is true of feelings and themes in our emotional lives. Clients will learn what some people have been doing and feel shame that they are not further along. Imagine if someone put you in the cockpit of a new 747 and told you to fly it! You have a basic idea of how planes work, but not a clue on even the first step. Now imagine a bunch of pilots watching you try.

This is what it is like for our clients. They have a general idea of how things should go, but they get overwhelmed as they have never been shown how. Teaching starts with giving them something different than what they already have been given and showing them how it can make a difference in how they feel. Help them understand that they may have been shown something unhealthy thousands and thousands of times.

I recently was visiting with a client with whom I had been making some progress. She grew up with a dad who abandoned her. Her mom who was an alcoholic and drug addict. Unfortunately, she was exposed to a number of harmful things during her abuse and neglect. She also had a step-father who was extremely verbally abusive, frequently telling her that she was worthless and not important. She shared that it was so bad that she had to leave the house.

In therapy, we identified that she clearly had the view that she was not important and did not matter. We progressed to a stage in which we were working on how things showed up in her everyday life. She shared one struggle in which the ringing of her business phone was prompting high anxiety and, at times, panic attacks. She said that she frequently changes her ring tones, as she begins to panic when she hears the same one over and over. She shared how she is fearful that when the phone rings, it is likely someone who is critical of something that she has done wrong, and they are calling to tell her about it.

This client also expressed that her home life was so miserable that she dropped out of school and took her GED so she could get to college more quickly. She went to college, graduated, and started her own business. She is clearly a hard-working, resilient, and successful person, but she does not *know* that or feel that.

Back to the phone call problem. I encouraged her to look at her phone-call anxiety form a different view and theme—one that expresses that she is okay, is loved, matters, and is successful. I told her to look at the phone calls coming into her office as coming from people who need her and are asking for help, as she has a particular skill set they lack. They need her!

Her face showed instant relief, and she said, "I have never thought of it that way." Here is someone who basically had no parental support and was told and shown many times that she was worthless. She raised herself, went to college, and started her own successful business, but she never thought of herself as someone who could be valuable. She was never taught that, and therefore never knew how that would even look. She comes into counseling seeking help for her anxiety issues, as she feels as though she is not successful and has no skills. As a therapist, giving someone a new set of skills to approach life is one of my most cherished rewards. I give this example to illustrate how important it is to help teach clients different responses, as they will not be able to see them themselves until we highlight these feelings and then provide some teaching.

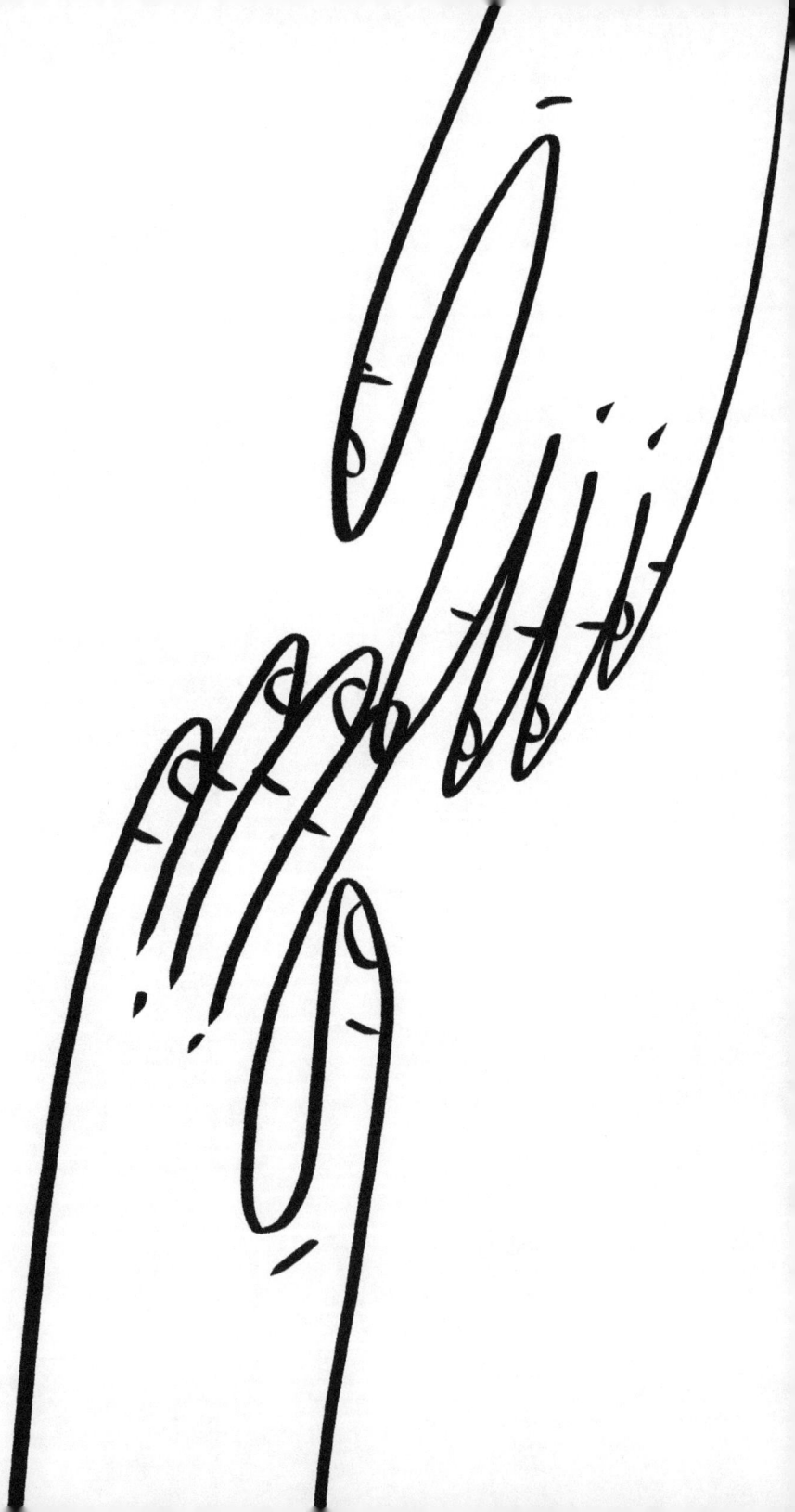

Getting stuck

GETTING STUCK

The process of helping clients become aware of their theme, identify when it is happening, and implement changes will work most of the time, but not all of the time. Unfortunately, we'll eventually encounter situations in which we're doing everything we can to try and help an individual or couple, yet the counseling will fail or get stuck. There are times when we get stuck in spots, and things can dramatically stall out. We need to step back and examine these moments, as if you can identify the cause, you can possibly help your client get out of the situation.

SCARED TO CHANGE

We can repeatedly talk in sessions about the need to change, but clients can often get stuck because they are afraid to change. They hear us, but the thought of doing something differently may be too scary to actually implement any type of change.

This can be difficult to identify, as they may be sitting in your office committed to counseling for a few sessions. They have been willing to talk about their situation, they've explored the old patterns of how they handled things, and they've even helped by identifying some good homework. But when they return to the office, they've failed to follow through on the homework and repeat the same dysfunctional patterns.

You have not met any resistance up until this point. If you feel as though you have a good connection and they seem engaged but are not making progress, this can be because they feel scared and are too afraid to do anything differently. One effective remedy is to help them verbalize and identify that they are scared. Ask them to reflect and examine their fear and express why they are afraid. What do they think will happen? Are they so afraid of failing, as in, "I don't want to take the chance that this might not work, because if it doesn't, I will be in a worse place than I am in right now." That fear, though illogical, can pretty powerful.

We often see an example of this in relationships. A woman will come in seeking help with trying to be more assertive and set healthy boundaries (the theme), and we will have discussed how to do things differently. The client will share a story of something that happened during the week and its effect. I will hear her share the feelings and how the incident impacted her. I will then ask, "What did your husband say when you said that?" She will reply, "Oh, I couldn't tell him that!" She did the homework with me, but not to her husband. I will then give her the assignment to go home and simply tell your husband what you just told me, and she will say, "I could not say that. I would not know how to do that."

I have often said, "Well if you do it just how you did it to me in the office, it will be fine." But the thinking that is going on behind the scenes that is not said out loud is this. "I can tell my husband, 'Hey if you are not too busy and you have time could you run and pick up the kids.' And if he says, 'No I am working in the garage,' I will be annoyed, but he was probably busy and had something more important."

That hurts her and even sends the message that she is not as important as the other things he may be doing, but she has left herself an out by forming it as a question and suggestion. So if he says no, it may be because of the reason she offered (too busy and have no time), which has nothing to do with her. The danger is that when you leave an out or make it vague, it will sometimes get missed. Obviously, the homework is to be assertive and share her feelings. The homework instructs her how to be clear and bold, stating something such as, "I am overwhelmed right now and you could really help me feel better and relieve some stress for me by getting the kids."

This is more direct and relays an accurate feeling of what she is experiencing at the time. However, notice that if he gives the answer of, "No I am working in the garage," he has really rejected her and there is no way to couch that answer with excuses. If she does this and that is his answer, she now has a bigger problem for which she can't make excuses, and she will have to face the fact that her husband does not want to meet her needs.

This fear is why an individual will often talk in sessions but not act outside of them. Helping clients to stop pretending that they are working on change is a way to help them get out of this situation. I will frequently remind clients that people don't pay counselors to help them stay the same. Repeatedly talking about how her husband does not show he cares and that she is not assertive or setting good boundaries does not help create change. By being assertive, even if it goes badly, she now has taken the next step in beginning to fix and address things with her husband.

NOT COMMITTED TO CHANGE

Fear is not the only reason people get stuck. As strange as it may sound, there are some people who do not want to get better. This type of client will talk about issues and be willing to look at problems without ever really wanting things to change—not for fear but for not wanting to change the status of the current situation. They may have come in stating that they did not like how things were going and wanted change, but in reality they are comfortable with their current situation and there is some type of pay-off or reward for the status quo.

They feel that if things would change, they would lose their identity or even their power. A client may have adopted their identity from their view of, "I am never heard"—kind of a martyr-type view that often tends to be more of a fatalistic perspective. You may hear a client say something like, "I am just doomed to do everything. He will never help me out." This perspective can provide an identity and a freedom to be frustrated, but it also allows her to not have to act, as this is her fate or perceived lot in life.

Let's look at the earlier example with the wife asking for help. If she says this in a bold way, and he listens and does go pick up the kids, she now has to respond differently and therefore loses her identify as the person whom no one helps. She may have to change her identity and do things that show that she loves her husband and appreciates his help. This is something different for which she may not be prepared. Taking away someone's perceived lot in life can be a change, and one they might not want to undertake. This provides a tough challenge for a therapist.

One option is to take a clear, almost confrontational approach of acceptance. Point out to the client that if they don't want to change, then maybe our job should switch and focus on how to help her cope with a husband who is uncaring. Help her accept her so-called lot in life. If this is how she sees her lot in life and she does not want to change, then the only other choice is to help her with acceptance—meaning nurture the view that this is how things are going to be, and the more time she spends lamenting only does a disservice to herself. She needs to learn how to not have his uncaring attitude affect her daily life.

This approach is similar to the paradoxical approach to change used in some therapy theories. Helping the client work hard to stay in the same spot can cause her to realize that perhaps it is worth the risk to change. This change-vs.-acceptance piece is really important and deserves some further explanation.

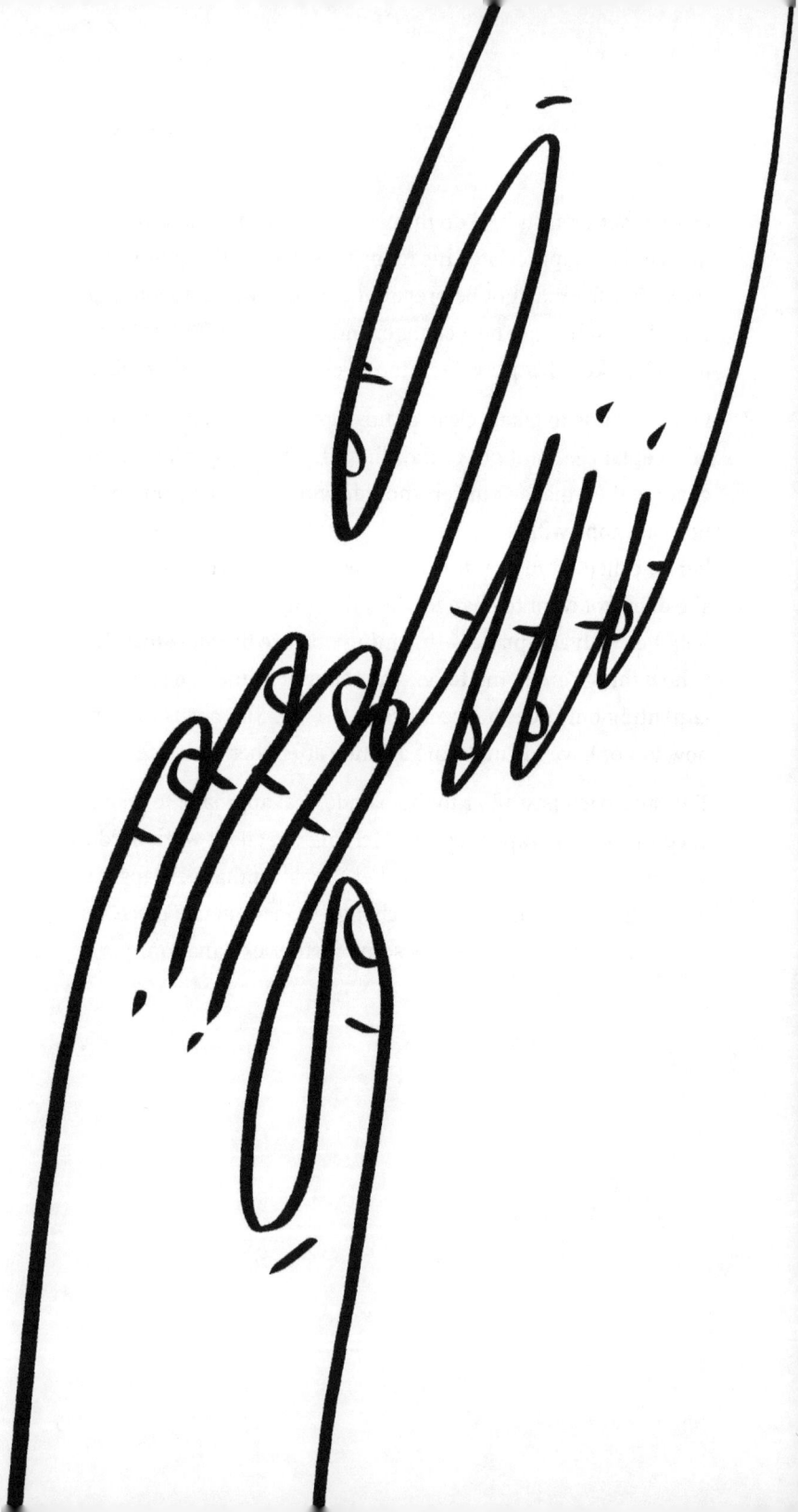

Acceptance vs. change

ACCEPTANCE VS. CHANGE

Even when we experience streaks of smooth sessions, there almost always comes a time in counseling when it gets really hard. Sessions might have been going okay, and your clients have been making some progress and discovered some insight into their situation. They may have even made a few changes in how they handle things. However, the day will come when we draw closer to what Aaron Beck calls the core beliefs that are the most difficult to change. (I highly recommend Beck's primer on cognitive behavioral therapy about the changing of beliefs.)

Your clients will eventually be challenged by tough decisions of not only do they want to change, but a realization of how hard that actually will be. It is one thing to change how they handle certain situations. It is a whole different thing to change how they view or perceive situations or life in general. That is the hard part. Clients will come to the crossroads of acceptance or change. You will hear it when they figure it out and verbalize their realization. Don't miss this, as it is a great time to review goals and remind them of why they are seeking help and guidance. You can miss these moments if you are not paying attention and you and your client are focused on specific problem solving that shadows the main issue. Here's an example of how this can present itself.

Therapist: "How did your visit go when you went down to see your mother?"

Client: "Well, I practiced what we talked about and I was less anxious for the first day. I was there, but then on the second day she started doing what she always does and started criticizing me on how I am raising my children. She always does this, sometimes so smoothly that I am not even aware of how often it is happening. I end up feeling guilty and feeling awful about myself. I just don't think that I can keep visiting her anymore."

Therapist: "Okay."

Client: "Are you saying that I don't have to visit her anymore? How is that okay? I need to honor my parents, don't I? My children need to have contact with their grandparents. I could never do that. My mother would be so angry at me, and besides, she would never let that happen, anyways!"

Notice all the questions that the client is sharing. This frequently happens when clients feel particularly anxious. She is worried about her current situation, as she is seeing that she may be stuck. In this scenario, the client is worried that that I am going to tell her that it is not worth it for her to have contact with her mother and she should just stop all contact. This is not what she wants.

This worry about what I may say or tell her to do when it is not what she wants comes from the connection between therapist and client. She values and cares about what I think of her. We have formed a connection, which means that the things I say will actually have some power and impact. She will listen and reflect on my perspective because there is a level of connection between us. It is important not to answer all the questions that are being fired at you, but you need to let her express the racing thoughts. They allow her to truly reflect on the idea of not having any contact with her mother and what that could potentially look like. Now with my personality, I will tend to not only let her reflect, but I tend to push the discussion a little further to get the client be a little more invested in the situation:

Therapist: "I am pretty sure your mother cannot make you have contact with her."

Client: "Well, you know what she is like." (*I have never met her and only "know" her through our conversations, but this is another small way that connection is illustrated*). "She does not quit until she gets her way."

Therapist: "Well, I guess you are stuck and are going to have to give into her way and feel crappy every time you visit her."

Client: "Well, that sucks. That is not really helpful. What am I supposed to do?"

Therapist: "Well you have two choices. We can work to help you learn how to accept the situation that you are in, or we can work to help you learn how to change the situation you are in. I can't pick for you (*client's right to self-determination*), as it your choice. I can even make it harder for you by adding that there is not a right choice in this situation! That is why you keep getting stuck, as there is no 'right' way to navigate this. But this struggle is part of the reason you struggle with your self-confidence and moods *(the real reason she came in for counseling)*. You are trying to do what you think is right by visiting your mother, and when you feel beat-up by doing what you think is right, you second-guess yourself. If you are doing what you think is the right thing and it is not working, you must have done something wrong if you are feeling this way. Repeat this pattern a number of times, and it has a negative effect on you. What do you think of that idea?"

I always ask for feedback when I make a guess on why someone acts or feels a certain way. That is a pretty big statement when I am trying to make the connections for her. I may be wrong, and I don't want to tell her how to feel. I want to ask her if I am correct in how I interpret her feelings. I also want to give her freedom to fine tune it, edit it, and make it better and more personal for her.

Client: "Well, I don't think I can keep going this way, so I have to do something differently."

The client has now really embraced that she needs to do something differently, and that she is not okay with simply accepting this situation. We've now reframed her issue in a way to help her improve her moods and self-esteem. If we were to go too quickly, it is really easy to just try a give her some coping skills on how to deal with her mother when she visits. Although these will be beneficial and important, they don't tackle the greater problem. To really help her, we need to frame it in a way that helps her understand that she is making significant life-changing steps when she is attacking how to deal with her mother. That is change!

Now here's the other half of the choice—acceptance. Acceptance is not often chosen in therapy, and when it is, therapy tends to finish quickly as there are not a lot of things on which we need to work. Acceptance here is simply staying the same and learning not to be so hurt by what is occurring around you. It is important to be open for clients to choose acceptance, even though it may not be the path you would choose. It is often necessary to let them know that despite how it may sound, it tends to be a perfectly acceptable path to choose. You may one day be asked to help a client learn to stay in the situation they have chosen, even if it is a spot in which you would not choose.

Helping a client with acceptance tends to focus more on helping them see that they are still making a choice and that they are not stuck. They simply have evaluated that the price of change is too costly, and they have decided that the current struggle with which they are living is a better option than change. Counseling typically concludes once you help them with this understanding, as there is no more needing to be addressed. Some clients will experience some significant relief when they come to that conclusion.

You need to be aware and pay attention, as clients will often change their minds without telling you. They may have already chosen acceptance as you spend significant time on changing things not knowing that the client has already accepted the situation. Consider this possibility if you are finding new ways to approach something yet meet resistance. It is important that when you see they have accepted change, you move forward by starting to bring up that this issue is solved and you are ready to move forward to something else or proceed with termination preparation. If the client again brings up the problem, you need to remind them that they chose to manage the situation in an acceptance form of coping yet are frustrated that things are not changing. Reminding them of their choice helps them see that they are not stuck. They chose this path. And if they don't like this choice, it's time to reexamine the costs for and against change. We need to be aware that even though we could never live in that situation, our client may be able to or even want to.

Change vs. acceptance is at the balance of all therapy. Most of the resistance and struggles that come from therapy are when clients realize this, and then subsequently realize that for anything different to happen they are going to have to change. Everyone knows change is hard. Get your clients to see that they are not stuck but have the power to change or accept their situations. They have that power. And when they are able to see how the change will benefit them and/or make them healthier, they may willingly take on the challenge. They need to take the time to look at the alternative and realize that it's one they cannot accept.

PERSONALITY DISORDERS

Therapy can also find itself stuck when you're trying to use insight-based therapies when dealing with individuals who have significant personality disorders such as Borderline Personality, Schizophrenia, Narcissism, Anti-Social, etc. (the Axis 2 diagnoses from the DSM-5).

Clearly, some level of insight is still needed to help a client identify his themes and behaviors and how they impact the individual and those around him. But as this is not an area of specialization that I have, I tend to refer these cases out to someone who focuses in those areas.

REFERRING OUT TO OTHER THERAPISTS

Let me take a quick moment here to share the importance of referring to other therapists. As a beginning therapist, this was one mistake I often made. I had the attitude that if someone came in with a problem, I would try to help them, even if I had no clue about their particular issue.

Although I think this eventually made me well-rounded, allowed me to see a variety of people, and helped my practice, I am not sure it was the best way to serve the client. I had the view that if I referred clients out to other therapists, it meant that I was not good enough (One of my themes that I have to be aware of!). Now having been in practice for some years, I am able to see that I have my areas of expertise and others have theirs, and it is not a reflection on my skills or being adequately qualified. When you recognize that a client does not fit with how you work or has an issue with which you are not qualified to handle, you can be most helpful and successful by referring that client to a better-suited therapist.

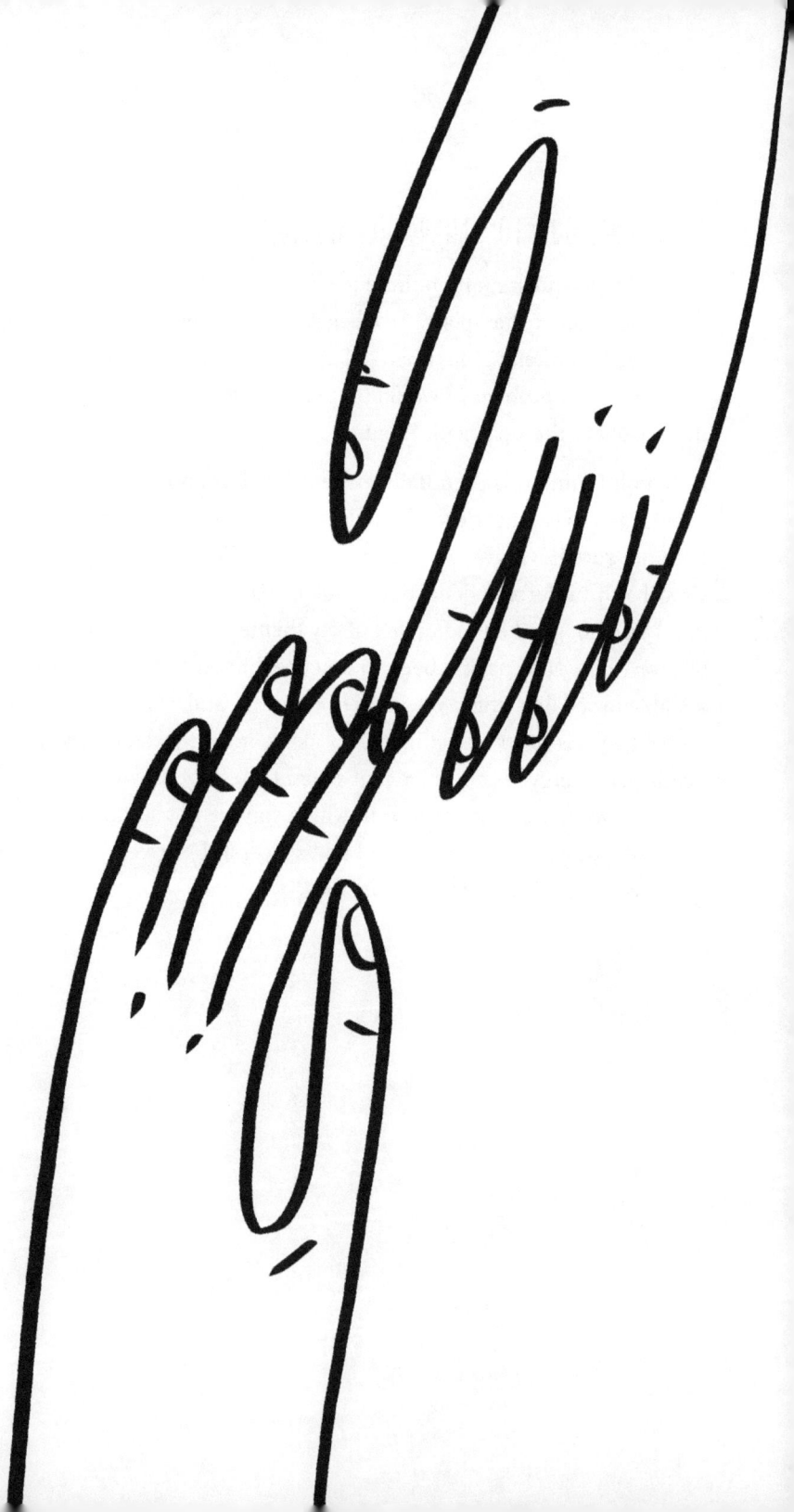

SECTION II: PART VI

Termination

TERMINATION

Finally, if you are successful with all the things we have talked about and your client successfully changes, feels better, and has been resolving things on their own, it is time to end therapy. Ending therapy with a client often does not go smoothly. In school, it always sounded as though you see someone for some sessions, and then both you and the client come to a conclusion that therapy is done. We have a celebration session in which we look back at the progress we have made, celebrate, and end the therapy.

That does not happen in real life very much. In my case, that is actually the least common scenario of how therapy ends. There are a number of ways therapy can end, and each one has an effect on you and your client. Let's look at a couple of these:

ONE AND DONE

This involves a client who comes in one time, and then you never see them again. I am not entirely sure why this is, as I am not able to follow up with them! If a client comes in and tells you too much, too quickly, they may be embarrassed and overwhelmed. This can happen when they have been struggling with something for quite a long time and finally get to the point in which they must deal with it. Often, they will even tell you, "This is the first time I have ever told someone this," or, "My husband and my parents don't even know this." This can be cathartic, but if the client talks too much, too quickly about how they feel, they may get some initial relief but will not prove beneficial in the long term. I have heard other counselors call it "emotional vomit," which actually makes a lot of sense. When you are sick to your stomach with the flu and you finally vomit, you do feel a big sense of relief. I think that this is very similar. After that initial relief passes, the client feels too vulnerable and exposed to come back to therapy. The treatment for this is to slow the client down and not let them unload too much, too quickly. This can be extremely hard to do. Can *you* puke slowly?

BRIEF, BUT INTENSE

This is typical with a client who is in some type of crisis. They come in and want another session right away. Sometimes, they feel as though they can't even wait a week. I typically see people every other week, or once a week if they are really struggling. They feel like they need to be seen twice in a week, as they need to figure out the crisis. Clients like this will come in as long as the crisis is intense. As soon as things settle down, they disappear. Unfortunately, they tend to treat the symptom and not the cause. They disappear at about the time the crisis abates and you were just getting ready to help them change so these crises don't happen again.

You can sometimes catch this potential during the initial assessment while reviewing their history, if you see that they have been to a number of different counselors over a period of time. This is pretty difficult to combat, as the client is usually not interested in long-term change or work. It's best to point out to them that you would like to help them learn how to change and manage their issues. Some will be able to slow down and look at the problem differently.

FADERS

In my experience, this is the most common way therapy ends. A client comes in, you and they do some great work, they make some changes over time, and they get healthy. How this looks from a session point of view is that they attend regularly every two weeks for a while. We then back it off to once every three weeks or once a month. When they come that first time after a month, we review how things are going and we talk about if they want to come back. Often, they are not quite ready to be done, so we schedule one in about a month. And when that time comes, they no-show the appointment. They've gotten better and gradually fade out of counseling.

There is nothing wrong with this, as long you have made sure that you have had your termination talk earlier in the sessions. I consider this type of termination to be the most normal in how they reflect real-life relationships. People grow, change, and move on with no distinct goodbye. Remember, we are trying to teach healthy, normal relationships, so why wouldn't our terminations be similar?

Think back to some of your relationships. Think of all the different friendships that you have had. How come you don't hang out with so-and-so anymore? What happened to that couple with whom you and your wife used to do things? Did you make a conscious effort to end that relationship and move on to other friends? Some friends last the test of time, and some come and go in our lives. We do not make conscious choices to end those relationships; they or you just grow in different directions. This is how I see most therapy relationships ending. The client becomes healthier and gradually moves away from sitting on your couch to a different place with a changed and healthier outlook.

TEXTBOOK

These are the clients who come in, participate in therapy, do the homework, acknowledge they are better, and then we decide to terminate together celebrate and they are gone! This does happen, but not often. These tend to be clients who are seeking help with a specific issue that has them stuck. They are able to identify when they have resolved or addressed the issue, and are totally comfortable with moving on and ending the therapeutic relationship in a healthy way. As I said, this does not happen often, but when it does it feels great from a therapist perspective. These are the clients who tend to thank you the most and are also able to verbalize the positive impact therapy had on their life.

CHANGE AND MAINTAIN

These clients are also some of my favorites, as you are able to establish a long-term relationship with them and you get to experience life along with them. These are clients who come in for a specific purpose or issue, and as it becomes resolved they identify the benefits therapy has had on them. They want to stay in therapy. Sometimes, we will change the focus to a new issue that they have identified and want to work on. When this happens, the change of focus is usually to something more personal. For example, a client may come in for help with parenting a child who has some struggles. Once that has settled down, the client sees some success. If you have built a relationship with her, you may hear something such as, "I feel like there are some other things that I want to work on. I had some bad things happen to me as a child and I would like to get past them. Do you do stuff like that, or do you only work with kids." This can present some challenges, as you fade out seeing one part of the family and increase seeing someone else, but that is the essence of family therapy—helping the family system. This situation again shows how important it is to make a connection with someone. Once it is made, clients are willing to go places and talk about things that they previously avoided.

Other clients might have no more issues but just want to keep coming. It is important if this happens to make sure you help clarify in the clients mind the new goals. It is helpful to help them understand that they have successfully changed their behaviors or feelings, and now we are simply doing maintenance or even preventive work. They need to know that they have succeeded at what they intended to do, and therapy does not need to last forever. They are capable. It's imperative here to make a clear distinction that we are moving into a different phase of therapy at their request. After making this distinction, sessions can take on a different look. The client may lead and tell you how they have addressed and handled new situations. The sessions tend to be spread out, sometimes months at a time, and can be are more reflective. Touching base periodically after helping something through a difficult time is pretty normal, and it speaks to both the connection you made and the difficulty of their journey.

No matter how therapy ends, it will end, and as mentioned earlier it usually does not end in a manner dictated by you the therapist. You have to be prepared for not always hearing the end of the story. Therapists frequently do not get to be a part of the happy ending. We get the honor and privilege to participate in the battle/struggle with them, but clients often go on to enjoy the victories without you. Learning how to feel satisfied with your role and not always knowing the outcome is something that all good therapists must learn if they want to continue practicing with a strong healthy outlook.

FIRING A CLIENT

Referring clients is one thing, but how about firing them? Have you ever had to tell a client that you could not work with them because you do not want to? I am a stubborn and tend not to give up, so I rarely do this. I actually think that I should do it more often. Recognizing that a connection cannot be made sounds like it negates everything we've discussed in this book, but firing a client can become necessary if you are not able to make a connection. It may be because of them, but it can also be because of you. First of all, it is important to realize that you can do this. You do have the right to be treated professionally. I have fired clients for attacking my staff or myself, causing damage or making scenes in the waiting room, too many no-shows, etc. It is hard to do as you, the therapist, can clearly see that they are hurting and in need of help, but setting healthy boundaries is as important for yourself as it is for your clients.

Conclusion

CONCLUSION

Well you made it to the end. Good job! Thanks for taking the time to go through this book. I hope you found it helpful. Remember, being a therapist is scary. You will have times in which you are lost and not sure what to do next. That is normal.

Remember the goal: You are trying to help people. To be able to help people, you need to be with people. Being with people and connecting with them can be costly and it can hurt, but that is how you help them. Remember, the theme of this book is to connect before anything else. People are unique and have a wide variety of challenges, but sometimes the biggest challenge is staying with them when they are lost and scared. If you can connect, everything else gets a little easier and you will be more successful at helping others.

I would love to hear your thoughts and feedback from this book. What have you learned? What things help you make connections with your clients? Please let me know. I would like a continued connection with you, the reader, so I, too, can grow!

About the Author

ABOUT THE AUTHOR

Tony Boer is a licensed clinical social worker in private practice. He has been practicing since 1998. He has worked in a variety of settings. Residential settings, hospitals, community agencies and private practice. He has also supervised a number of students learning how to help effectively.

He can be reached at: Tonyboer.secc@midconetwork.com.

www.ingramcontent.com/pod-product-compliance
Lightning Source LLC
Chambersburg PA
CBHW022333280326
41934CB00006B/619